Be Your Own BEAUTICIAN

—the complete solution to your body and beauty problems unfolded by a renowned beautician

Parvesh Handa
Beautician and Cosmetologist

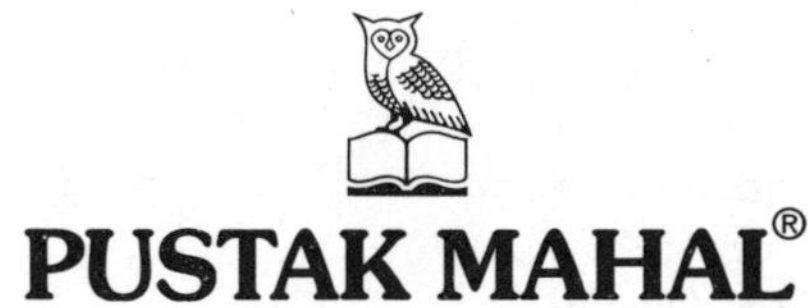

PUSTAK MAHAL®

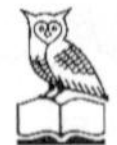
Publishers
Pustak Mahal®

J-3/16 , Daryaganj, New Delhi-110002
☎ 23276539, 23272783, 23272784 • *Fax:* 011-23260518
E-mail: info@pustakmahal.com • *Website:* www.pustakmahal.com

Sales Centre

- 10-B, Netaji Subhash Marg, Daryaganj, New Delhi-110002
  ☎ 23268292, 23268293, 23279900 • *Fax:* 011-23280567
  E-mail: rapidexdelhi@indiatimes.com
- **Hind Pustak Bhawan**
  6686, Khari Baoli, Delhi-110006
  ☎ 23944314, 23911979

Branches

Bengaluru: ☎ 080-22234025 • *Telefax:* 080-22240209
E-mail: pustak@airtelmail.in • pustak@sancharnet.in
Mumbai: ☎ 022-22010941, 022-22053387
E-mail: rapidex@bom5.vsnl.net.in
Patna: ☎ 0612-3294193 • *Telefax:* 0612-2302719
E-mail: rapidexptn@rediffmail.com
Hyderabad: *Telefax:* 040-24737290
E-mail: pustakmahalhyd@yahoo.co.in

© Author

ISBN 978-81-223-0973-7

Edition: 2011

The Copyright of this book, as well as all matter contained herein (including illustrations) rests with the Author. No person shall copy the name of the book, its title design, matter and illustrations in any form and in any language, totally or partially or in any distorted form. Anybody doing so shall face legal action and will be responsible for damages.

Printed at : **Unique Colour Cartoon, Delhi**

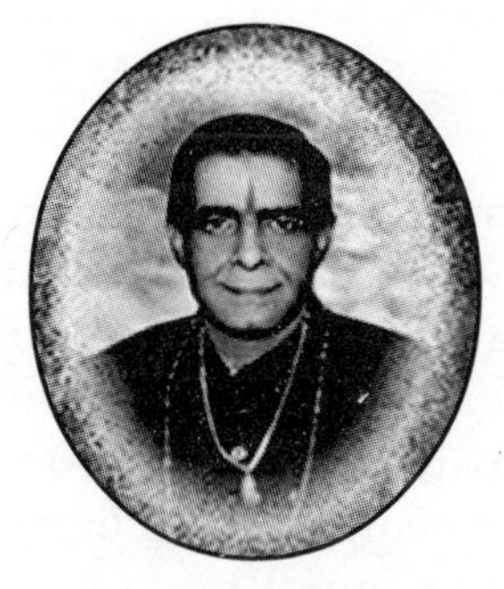

Lovingly dedicated to

Respected Guru Dev

Dr. Pt. Manmohan Shastri Ji

of Babyal, Ambala Cantt.

for his constant Gifts of Light, Life, Inspirations

&

Divine True Love

Preface

Beauty is a gift of Nature to men and women and it takes it away if neglected. Even the best-textured skin tends to face problems if not cared for properly. Body in totality makes for an attractive personality and it is essential to take regular care of each part of the body, from head to heel. This book deals with a 100 contemporary techniques which enhance beauty of skin, face and body.

The concept of beauty has widened in the last three decades. For achieving success in career, looks and guts are needed. It is seen that many men and women have the aptitude but not having proper knowledge, they are unable to get good results. The art of Indian make-up and hairstyles has no parallels. Indian faces are exotic enough without being too ethnic. Indian girls are smart and beautiful. They have lovely skin tones and natural looks. If they are assisted and well groomed, they are as good as the best in the world.

Glamour is not out of reach if one is fully conversant with correct techniques of living and know-how about what to wear, eat, and the art of make-up, so one can even match the famous glamorous women in the world. A survey conducted in this regard reveals that women, whether living in metros or in villages, have a penchant for glamour, beauty and fashion – but their hopes are not always fulfilled due to lack of knowledge and guidance.

You will find this book, although not too comprehensive in size, has touched all vital aspects to make you a self-confident, perfect, beautiful, glamorous person by describing dress sense, art of make-up, keeping hair and skin healthy, diet and exercising, personal hygiene and body care to self-grooming.

I hope this book will prove to be a good friend, a helping hand and a sincere advisor to all those (not only women but also men) suffering from disorders of skin and hair, which are curable with a little care, and save them from ailments later in life. I have tried to give maximum natural remedies based on herbal formulations in this book. Such remedies were unknown to Indian women decades ago. However, this awareness has increased rapidly in past over two decades and today the picture is different. Beauty-conscious people themselves have re-discovered the potential hazards of synthetic products and are shifting to natural products.

I am thankful to *Dr. D.S.Jaspal*, Patron & President, Indian Medical Association (Haryana) and *Dr. (Ms) Rita Jaspal,* Chairperson of IMA (Haryana), for the cooperation and assistance rendered to me for making this book useful to the readers, especially to those suffering from serious skin ailments.

I hope this book will help readers to avoid, control and cure their sufferings with a little care and timely treatment. The readers should keep in mind that medical treatments described in this book are a reference only, not a medical guide or manual for self-treatment. No medical treatment should be taken without consultation of a qualified doctor.

—Parvesh Handa

Contents

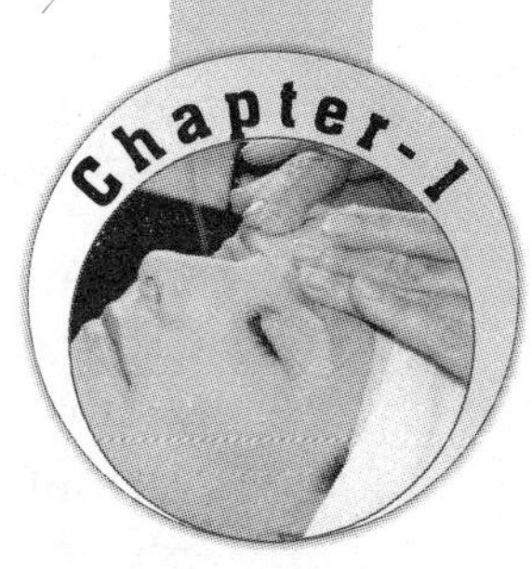

Advance Facial Techniques

Foundation of good skin

1. *Family Matters*: Family habits matter almost as much as genes. So when you are scanning your parent's faces, look at the furrows, nose to mouth lines and shape of the mouth. You have a tendency to move your face in the same way. Facial exercises can help put this right.
2. *Let it Breathe*: You need to breathe, and so does your skin. 7% of the oxygen you take into your lungs is used directly by your skin. Breathing in supplies your cells with essential oxygen, breathing out removes carbon dioxide (which would poison cells if left long enough) and waste from your body.
3. *Fresh Air*: Fresh air keeps your skin looking blooming. The benefit of walking by the sea, in a park full of trees or in the mountains is strikingly different from a walk along a crowded city.
4. *Carry on Moving*: Regular exercise is essential to the overall good health and functioning of our mind and bodies. When you exercise, oxygen surges to every cell in your body, allowing nutrients to be absorbed more efficiently and cells to grow faster. This means more collagen production, which leads to improved texture and moisture retention and a thicker, more resilient dermis. Aerobic exercise–brisk walking, jogging, running, bicycling, swimming or dancing will stimulate the circulation, prompt a sluggish digestion to eliminate wastes and toxins and bring an instant glow to your skin.
5. *Feed your Skin*: Some dermatologists dismiss the food you eat as if it couldn't affect the general state of your skin, although few could deny the connection between specific foods and skin reaction, from rashes and itching to eczema. We cannot deny that a diet rich in fresh foods—particularly fruits, vegetables and grains—and low in processed and refined foods will benefit your whole system including the skin.

   Eat plenty of:

   - Fresh fruits and vegetables, especially green and orange ones (including avocado and apples).
   - Dried fruits, cereals, pulses and grains.
   - A few eggs weekly, if you are non-vegetarian.
   - Oils, such as olive, sesame, walnut, hazelnut, safflower and sunflower.
   - Dairy products, wheat-germ, whole wheat bread and brown rice.

- Soya products.
- If you are non-vegetarian, have organic meat and fish.

6. *Sleep*: Scientists now believe that skin cells regenerate as we sleep, and it is one of the greatest free beautifiers. We also have a theory that a sound sleep relaxes our facial skin, so that lines and furrows are softened by the morning.
7. *Water*: Drink at least 1.5 litre of water a day. Tap water is definitely better than nothing. Experts advise that room temperature water is most compatible with your body. Spraying your face with spring water can make it dewy fresh on a hot day. Also try spraying after cleansing but before moisturising.

Ageing

Why does skin age? In a nutshell, it occurs as collagen and elastin, the two major components in the underlying support structure of the skin degenerate. The major factors in this degeneration are ultra violet (UV) light from the sun and damage by nasty molecules called free radicals. Both UV light and free radicals cause the collagen fibres to twist and the skin begins to line, sag and wrinkle. Exposure to the sun's rays can be avoided, since it causes much of the harm before the age of 18. Start using a sun preparation early and make sure your children do too to save the skin damage. From the age of 50, the number of elastin fibres declines tremendously, accelerating the droopping, bagging and sagging. At the same time, the skin becomes drier because oil production diminishes, as does the skin's ability to hold water, and the rate of cell renewal also reduces. By giving the skin some extra tender or loving care, however, makes your skin to respond quickly and positively.

Insufficient flow of sebum from the sebaceous glands makes the skin dry. For effective results, apply a negative galvanic electric current for 3 to 5 minutes. Exposure of face and neck to infrared lamp up to 5 minutes provides better results and closes the skin pores. Keep an infrared lamp about 24 inches away from the face. For dry skin, avoid using lotions which contain a large percentage of alcohol. Apply lubricating oil or eye cream over and under the eyes. The procedure for facial will be similar to the plain facial.

Skin facts

- The average adult has some 300 million skin cells, covering up to 2 sq. m. (about 21 sq. ft.) of the skin, weighing 3.2 kg.
- The facial skin is about 0.12 mm (0.005 in.) thick; body skin about 0.6 mm (0.02 in.); and the thickest area on the palms and soles about 1.2 mm (0.05 in.) or more up to 4.7 mm (0.09 in.).
- The thinnest skin is on the lips and eyes.
- Each square half inch of skin contains, on average, at least 10 hair, 100 sweat glands, 1 m. (3.2 ft.) long row of tiny blood vessels and 15 sebaceous glands.

How to analyse your skin before facial

Analyse your skin before the facial treatment. Remove make-up completely and sit before a mirror to determine the following:

- If the skin of your face is dry or oily?
- If the blackheads or acne are present?
- If broken capillaries are visible?
- If the texture of the skin is soft and velvety or harsh and rough?
- The type of face you have?

How to recognise your skin

Generally, the facial skin is classified into three different types:

1. **T-Zone:** This comprises the part of the forehead, the nose and the lips that are always oily.
2. **C-Zone:** This includes the part of the cheeks that are usually dry and sensitive, when there is redness in these parts.
3. **Y-Zone:** This is the area on the neck and the upper part of the chest.

This analysis will determine the choice of the creams and face packs to be used for massaging, the amount of pressure to be applied when doing a massage and the type of make-up to be applied after the facial and the areas on the face that need extra care.

Benefits of facial treatments

The hairstyle of a female may be very attractive and beautiful, but if the face that it frames is covered with an unattractive skin, it will reduce the beneficial effects of good grooming. Facial treatments are beneficial for the following reasons:

- To cleanse the skin.
- To increase circulation.
- To activate glandular activity.
- To relax the nerves.
- To maintain the muscle tone.
- To strengthen the muscle tissue.
- To correct skin disorders.
- To prevent formation of wrinkles and ageing lines.
- To soften and improve skin texture and complexion.
- To give a youthful look and feeling.

Essential points in facial massage

- Feel thoroughly relaxed when having facial.
- The atmosphere should be quiet (except light music) and clean.
- Follow a systemic procedure.
- If hands are cold, warm them before touching the facial skin.
- Make sure that the fingernails are not too long or pointed.
- Sponge face with cotton pledgets moistened with astringent lotion.
- Apply muscle oil around the eyes and neck if needed. Use lanolin or hormone cream for dry skin and cold cream for an oily skin.
- Remove ornaments before facial routine and if convenient, undress yourself and wear least possible clothes.

Quick home facial (30 minutes)

- Tie your hair away from face and neck and wear a bandeau.
- Cleanse your face and neck with a cleansing lotion and wipe off with a facial tissue.
- Apply cream all over the face in dots and blend it thoroughly, massaging your face and neck upwards.
- Steaming is an excellent way to revive your skin, stimulate the circulation and unclog the blocked pores of the skin. The process is known as **sauna facial.** Steam should be taken by leaning over a large bowl of boiling water and covering your head with a towel making a tent around the bowl of boiling water. Extract blackheads.
- Lie on your back when you have a face pack. Let it dry for 15-20 minutes, then wash off with lukewarm water.
- If your skin is dry, steam your face once a week. In case of excessively oily skin, steaming can be done daily.
- Do not go too close to the boiling water. If the steam is too hot, it might cause broken veins.

Facial for dry skin (45–60 minutes)

A dry skin is caused by an insufficient flow of sebum (thick oil secreting from the sebaceous glands). This facial assists in correcting the dry condition of the skin. It may be given with or without applying an electric current. Electric current is applied for more effective results. The procedure of a facial for dry skin is as following:

- Prepare for a plain facial. Apply cleansing cream, then remove with the tissue.
- Sponge face with cleansing lotion if the skin is dry.
- Apply negative galvanic current for 3-5 minutes (optional step).
- Apply emollient cream on the face.
- Apply muscle oil or eye cream over and under the eyes. Cover eyes with cotton pads moistened with witch-hazel or boric acid solution.

- Apply muscle oil over the neck.
- Give manipulations for three to five minutes. The faradic or sinusoidal current may also be used (optional step).
- Remove cream with tissue or warm moist towel.
- Apply skin lotion suitable for dry skin. The positive galvanic current may also be applied for a better result.
- Blot face with tissue or towel.
- Apply base foundation and make-up suitable for the skin tone.

***Precaution*:** For dry skin avoid the use of lotions which contain large percentage of alcohol.

Facial for dry, scaly skin with high-frequency current

The procedure for this kind of facial is similar as described above, except giving manipulations using the indirect method of applying the high-frequency current for not more than 5-7 minutes.

Facial for oily skin (50-60 minutes)

An oily skin has blackheads due to improper diet consisting of too much starchy and oily food. Blackheads are formed by a hardened mass of sebum in the ducts of sebaceous glands.

- Prepare for a plain facial.
- Apply cleansing cream. Remove with warm, moist towel. If the skin is excessive oily it may be washed with warm water and medicated soap.
- Apply cleansing lotion for oily skin.
- Apply negative galvanic current for not more than 3-5 minutes to open pores or steam the face with the facial steamer to open pores.
- Gently press out blackheads (do not press hard enough to bruise the skin tissue) with fingertips covered with tissue or blackhead extractor.
- Sponge the face with an antiseptic.
- Apply blue light over the bare skin for not more than 3-5 minutes.
- Apply massage cream suitable for an oily skin and give manipulations.
- Use faradic current, if possible.
- Remove cream with warm, moist towel.
- Prepare a cotton pledget moistened with an astringent lotion and apply to the face and neck with upward and outward movement to close the pores or apply positive galvanic current for less than 5 minutes to close pores.
- Blot excess moisture with tissue.
- Apply base foundation and a suitable make-up.

Facial for oily skin with whiteheads

Whiteheads (Milia) is a common skin disorder formed by sebaceous matter, and usually occurs within or under a fine texture skin. Because of small surface openings, the sebum cannot excide and collects in small, hardened, round, pearly white formations under the skin, which can be drained out by a dermatologist.

Facial for acne skin (60 minutes)

Acne being a disorder of the sebaceous glands requires medical direction by the cosmetologist to reduce the oiliness of the skin by local applications, removing blackheads with a sanitised blackhead extractor, cleansing the skin, using specialised medicated cosmetic preparations and suggesting regulated diets discouraging acne. The procedure for facial for acne treatment is as following:

- Cleanse face with medicated soap and warm water or a towel wrung out of hot water and medicated soap.
- Apply acne cream or ointment over face and neck.
- Apply the high-frequency current with direct application over the affected parts for not more than 5 minutes.
- Remove the acne cream or ointment with tissues or warm moist towel.
- Apply thick cotton mask to the affected parts on the face saturated with acne lotion. Retain for 10 minutes.
- Remove mask and blot residue with cool, wet towel.
- Saturate cotton pledgets with astringent lotion, applying with a light blotting movement.
- Moisten a piece of cotton with an antiseptic lotion and touch each pimple or acne.
- Clean up the facial skin. Avoid using make-up, if possible.

Role of diet in case of skin prone to acne and pimples

A faulty diet is one of the common causes of acne. Avoid foods high in fats, starches and sugars, which make acne worse. Avoid eating sweets, creams, fried foods, butter, white bread, potato chips, whole milk, ice cream, chocolate and fat meats.

Hot oil mask facial for a skin prone to wrinkles (50-60 minutes)

A hot oil mask facial is recommended for a dry, scaly skin prone to wrinkles. The following formula for hot oil mask is suggested. Mix the following ingredients:

Olive Oil	2 tablespoons
Castor Oil (Refined grade)	1 tablespoon
Glycerine	1/4 teaspoon

Procedure:

- Give a plain facial, including removal of emollient cream.
- Moisten gauze with warm oil and place on the face, starting at the throat.

- Cover eyes with eye pads.
- Place an infra-red lamp about 24 inches from the face for 5-10 minutes.
- Remove gauze.
- Apply emollient or moistening cream.
- Give facial manipulations, followed by applying warm steam towel.
- Apply astringent lotion and light make-up.

Facial for a sensitive and dehydrated skin (50 minutes)

It is also known as vitamin C facial. The procedure is similar to a plain facial as below:

- Cleansing with cream, milk or lotion according to the type of skin.
- Apply a skin food according to the skin type, followed by lymphatic massage manipulations for about 10 minutes.
- Apply peeling face mask, followed by application of vitamin C fluid on the face with light friction.
- A high frequency treatment is recommended in case of severely dehydrated and sensitive skins.

Facial for muscle toning treatment

This treatment is designed to produce a more vigorous effect on the deeper tissues and muscles. Muscle toning (muscle strapping) is very beneficial for the older women whose face and neck show tendency to sag, in case of a flabby face and neck (due to illness), appearance of a double chin and heavy jowls and solid deposits of fatty tissue on the face causing flabbiness. The following procedure is applied:

- Apply cleansing cream. Remove cream with warm moist towel.
- Apply cleansing lotion, followed by application of emollient cream.
- Steam the face with a facial steamer or warm towels. Remove blackheads, if necessary and sponge face with an antiseptic.
- Re-apply emollient cream. Also apply cream around, over and under the eyes.
- Pat on muscle oil and give special massage manipulations gently using hands (slightly cupped) and fingers (middle and ring fingers). Be careful as these tissues are delicate and bruise easily.

Oxygen bath facial treatment for post-acne skin (50-60 minutes)

It is suitable for young and matured skins. The following steps are suggested for this facial treatment:

- Cleanse the skin with cream or milk. Remove cream with warm moist towel.
- Suction with softening milk.
- Steam the face for 3-5 minutes for opening the skin pores.

- Apply vitamin cream on oily skin and mint gel on a dry skin.
- Massage for 10-15 minutes.
- Apply oxygen-rich mask for 15 minutes, which heals the damaged acne.
- High frequency treatment up to 5 minutes in severe cases.
- Sometimes, after the facial treatment a couple of acne appear on the face, which is a good sign.

Facial for ageing, wrinkled and dry skin (45-50 minutes)

- Cleanse with cream, milk or lotion.
- Massage with cream for 15 to 20 minutes.
- Apply Thermo-herb pack.
- Extract blackheads.
- Apply cold compression.
- Also apply sun protection cream.

Vegetable peeling mask (45 minutes)

This facial treatment is most beneficial for oily skin without pimples and acne, and is in seven stages as described below:

- Cleansing skin of the face and the neck with rose water.
    - High frequency (HF) or ozone treatment is the second stage of this facial treatment. HF is characterised by a high rate of oscillation, or vibration. It is commonly called the violet ray or alkaline rays used for both scalp and facial treatments. The HF may be used to treat thin hair, itchy scalp, excessive oily or dry skin. The primary action of this current is thermal or heat producing. Because of its rapid vibration, there are no muscular contractions. The physiological effects are either stimulating or soothing, depending on the method of application. The electrodes for high frequency are made of glass or metal in flat or round shape. As the current passes through the glass electrodes, tiny violet sparks are emitted. The treatment should start with a mild current and gradually increase to the required strength. There are two methods of applying the HF current: *Direct Surface Application* (recommended for acne-prone or oily skin) and *Indirect Application* (the skin is covered with gauge before applying the HF current).

The high frequency treatment has the following benefits:

1. Stimulates circulation of blood.
2. Increases glandular activities.
3. Aids in elimination and absorption.
4. Increases metabolism.

5. Leaves germicidal action when used.
6. Relieves congestion.
7. Turns acidic skin to dry skin tone.
8. Helps in removing blackheads and whiteheads.
9. Controls sebaceous glands.
10. Increases water level in young skins lacking oil.

Caution: High frequency current should not be used on the pregnant, asthmatic, those suffering from high blood pressure, patients of sinus blockage or metal implants, if the skin is dehydrated or wrinkled or swollen and itchy.

- Apply vegetable peel pack when the skin is semi-dry.
- Apply medicated cream. Leave for 5-7 minutes and rub with a brush applying fruit juice or cucumber juice or raw milk.
- Remove blackheads with blackhead extractor.
- After cold compression, apply sun protection cream.

Alpha Hydroxy Acid (AHA) treatment facial (45 minutes)

This facial treatment is recommended for fairness and all types of skins. The procedure of this facial treatment is as following:

- Cleanse the skin with a cleansing cream, milk or lotion.
- Suction with the help of a softening milk.
- Application of alkaline scrub (optional).
- Face steaming and friction massage (or lymphatic massage) for 15-20 minutes with cream (mixture of skin food and gel), followed by removing blackheads.
- To remove infection use high frequency and a protein mask (if the skin is oily and prone to acne)
- If the skin is sensitive, apply whitening mask instead of the AHA mask for 20-30 minutes.

Under eye dark circles treatment (30-45 minutes)

Dark circles under the eyes appear because of the following reasons:

- Salt in the tears that turns area around eyes black.
- Continuous flow of water from eyes.
- Low diet.
- Loss of water in the body.
- Damaged capillaries.

Procedure: Wear gloves before starting the treatment. Clean the eyes. Before starting the treatment give a face touch, instead of touching the relaxing eyes. For eye treatment, products

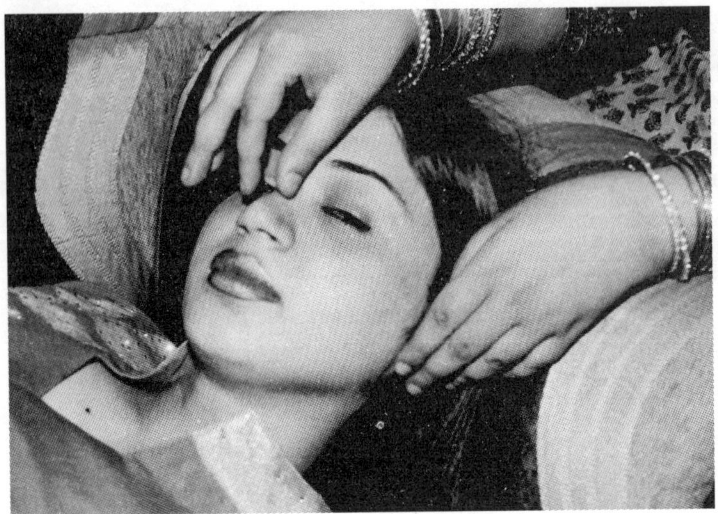

such as fish, oil, collagen water (or rose water), mint gel, skin food (AHA mask) are required. For eye treatment, gently start giving suction from inside towards the outside direction. Clean the eyes. Apply the AHA mask on the area around the eyes. Cover lobes (round flat projecting part of eye) with warm cotton dipped in rose water. Give steam to the facial skin for a little while. Massage the area around the eyes gently not more than two minutes. A high frequency current can be applied for 2-3 minutes.

Wrinkles under the eyes

The skin around the eyes is very fine and delicate and it tends to dry out very quickly. From 25 years onwards, occasionally apply a little eye cream or special eye oil to counteract dryness around the eyes. Do not rub your eyes if there is irritation or burning, otherwise the skin will shrink and wrinkles will appear on it. To avoid such wrinkles, use anti-wrinkle cream or almond oil. Here are a few home recipes:

- Boil water with leaves of the tea and filter. Soak a cotton swab in it and foment the area around the eyes daily until you get satisfactory results.
- Wrinkles and lines are the first to form on the face but they are not caused by age. They are caused by expression and as such are known as laughter lines. The upward slanting laughter lines are attractive and give character to a face. The downward sloping angular lines caused by tension, worry and anxiety are less pleasing.
- Always massage slowly with oil or cream with fingers the area around the eyes and remove the surplus oil or cream after 30 minutes, otherwise your eyes will become puffy.
- Lack of sleep results in dark rings below the eyes and sometimes the skin becomes flabby. An eight-hour rest in a day keep the eyes healthy.

Pouches and dark shadows around the eyes

The skin around the eyes is the most sensitive because the hypodermis, which exists everywhere else, is lacking here. Let the eyes get plenty of rest. An adult needs minimum eight hours sleep during the day (in 24 hours) whereas a child needs 12 hours sleep.

Puffy eyes

Puffy eyes may be the sign of something wrong with your general health, but if your doctor says there is nothing wrong then check whether you are using too rich and nourishing cream for your eyes and leaving it on all night. Wipe off the cream after 15 to 20 minutes. To add sparkle to the eyes, put ten chamomile (babuna plant) flowers into ½ litre of boiling water. When it cools, dab your eyes with this solution using a wet pad.

European facial (40 to 50 minutes)

It includes easy-to-follow, step-by-step procedures and routines such as extensive facial massage, use of sponges to clean the skin and remove stale make-up, applying cream and moisturiser, steaming the face, exfoliation, extracting blackheads, applying face pack and to remove the mask.

Express facial (25 minutes)

The facial steps comprise relaxation, cleansing, warm compresses, soothing massage, nourishing, herbal extracts which leave the skin revitalised and moisturised.

Classic facial (50 minutes)

This facial helps to begin the balancing process for your skin. The facial routine includes deep pore cleansing, exfoliation to remove the dull surface of the skin cells, gentle extractions to remove deeper impurities and application of a mask that will benefit your exact skin type and specific needs.

Anti-ageing facial (50 minutes)

It is a unique combination of powerful anti-oxidation and nourishing essential oils which leave the delicate skin velvety smooth and supple. This facial is ideal for sensitive or environmentally-stressed skin types.

Hydraderm facial (30 minutes)

It is a high-tech skin therapy which makes the use of mild electrical currents that leave the skin deeply cleansed, hydrated, regenerated and oxygenated. The results of this treatment are excellent, immediate and long lasting.

Hydradermine lightening treatment (30 minutes)

This facial is a beauty treatment with visible, lasting results promoting fresh skin. In this facial, active lightening ingredients are diffused by gentle ionisation to procure a radiant, clear, visibly lighter and even complexion.

Aroma facial–a holistic therapy (50 minutes)

Aroma facial consists of eight steps: cleansing, natural refreshing tonic, herbal compress, essential oil massage, application of compress or poultice, facial mask, application of moisturisers and rest. The process of cleansing is to thoroughly remove from the skin all traces of make-up and other products such as general dirt and grime. Certain essential oil components have the capacity not only to penetrate the epidermis and dermis but enter the bloodstream. Even the cleanest-looking skin needs cleansing to get rid of the atmospheric pollution. Apply gently the cleanser over the face and the throat. Now remove the cleanser with the toner. Choose a base oil according to the type and condition of the skin. Essential oil helps to revitalise the face, making it feel refreshed, relaxed, energised and relieves stress and tension. If using a poultice or compress, this is the stage to apply. Now apply facial mask, rinse off when it dries, then apply the moisturiser. Rest for few minutes in the end. Use a pure natural moisturiser. Do not add essential oil to this. Essential oils such as Palmarose, Rose, Jasmine, Geranium, Tangerine and Chamomile Roman relax the body. When massaged during pregnancy, these prepare the body for an easier delivery.

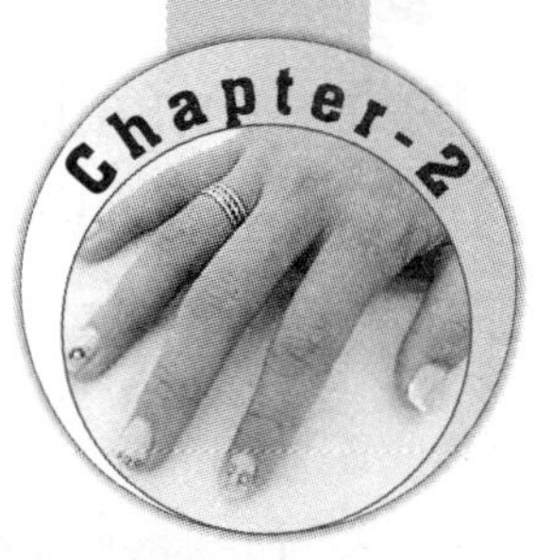

Manicure, Pedicure and Depilation

Manicure is a Latin word. 'Mani' means hand, 'cure' means care. Taking care of hands, fingers and nails is called *Manicure.* If there is any pus on the sides of the nails or cuts, boils, burns or an infection, manicure should not be done. In case suffering from cold, cough and fever, avoid manicure. The following steps should be undertaken:

- Remove the old nail polish with cotton wool soaked in a remover. Now file your nails in an oval shape, file towards the tip and never deep down the nail, as this will weaken the nail.
- Now soak your fingers in warm soapy water for five minutes. Add a pinch of borax or oat flour to give extra softness. Use a nail brush to clean the nails. Lukewarm solution may contain shampoo, hydrogen peroxide (H_2O_2)—½ teaspoon each and a few drops of Dettol.
- Clean under the nails with cotton tipped orangewood stick. If the nails become hard while filing, dip them in tepid oil to keep them soft. Do not dip fingers in oil before filing because the nail gets brittle and breaks.
- Apply cuticle remover with a nail pusher. Apply cuticle cream and massage into the nails. Wash and apply base coat or a colourless nail varnish. Let it dry, then apply the second coat. Rubbing lemon peel is effective for ensuring strong nails.

Do's and don'ts while manicuring

- Sharp, pointed implements should be handled with care.
- Be careful not to drop implements on the floor.
- Do not file too deeply into the nail corners.
- Do not use a sharp, pointed implement to cleanse the under nail.
- Use emery board on the over-sharp edges of the implements.
- Apply an antiseptic immediately if the skin is accidentally cut.
- Never push the cuticle back too far.
- Apply septic powder to stop bleeding from a small cut.
- Avoid too much pressure at the base of the nail.
- Abstain from working on a nail that is diseased or contains pus.

Deluxe manicure

The steps include bleaching, normal manicure, vibratory massage and hand pack.

1. **Bleaching:** 20 minutes

   Mix 2 teaspoons of hydrogen peroxide, 1 teaspoon of ammonia and 2-3 teaspoons of kaolin powder.
2. Massage and perform the normal manicure.
3. **Vibratory Massage:** 2-3 minutes.
4. **Hand Pack:** 30 minutes.

   Mix 3 teaspoons of each: almond oil, olive oil and til oil, 1 egg yolk, 2 teaspoons of honey and kaolin powder or *besan.* Apply this pack on hands. When dry, wash it off. Rinse in vinegar water to remove the smell of egg.

Super deluxe manicure

It is also called as *oil manicure.* Bleaching is not done in super deluxe manicure. Take ½ cup of almond oil. Dip your fingers in lukewarm almond oil for 10-15 minutes.

Give steam under a hot towel to the hands. Apply hand pack for 10-15 minutes. Thermo-herb pack can be applied for wrinkles and aged skin. Remove the pack with lukewarm water. Now apply a moisturiser. Apply nail varnish or nail paint.

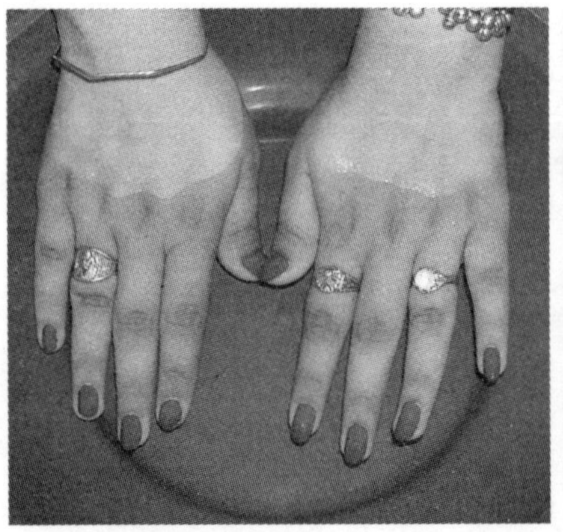

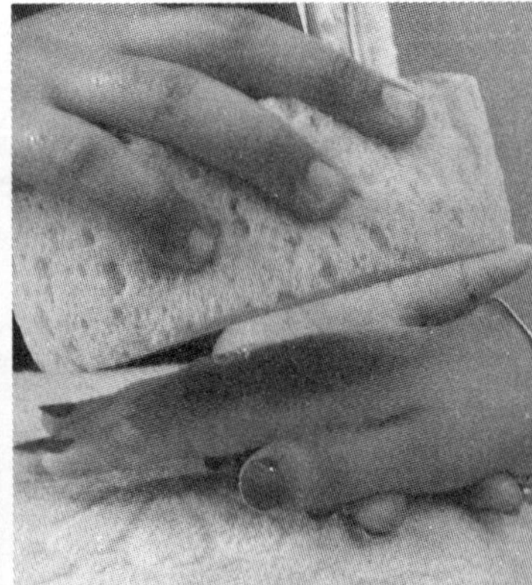

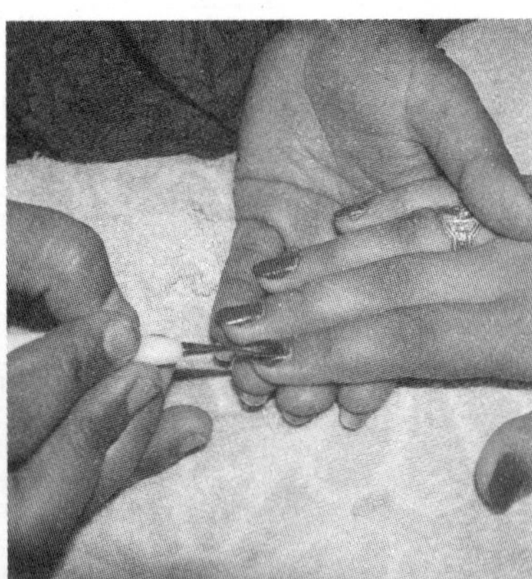

Oil manicure

An oil manicure is particularly beneficial for ridged and brittle nails. It keeps the skin of the hands soft and pliable. The following remedies are suggested:

1. Use coconut oil. Warm the oil to a comfortable temperature before use.
2. Place fingers in the warmed oil for 30 to 60 seconds according to the condition.
3. Massage the hands and wrists with oil. Now remove oil from the hands.

4. Apply skin freshener. The nails should be wiped carefully with polish remover to remove all traces of oil before applying nail polish.
5. All other operations are similar to a plain manicure.

Men's manicure

Generally men prefer a conservative manicure. The nails are filed either in round or square shape. A dry polish is used, which is available only at selective cosmetic stores in big cities. The implements, material and supplies are the same as those used for a general manicure.

Buffing of nails

The nails are buffed with an application of a small amount of powder polish over the buffer. It increases the circulation of the blood to the fingertips, smoothes the nails and gives them a natural gloss or polish. Where a clear or neutral liquid polish is to be applied, remove the powder polish particles by washing and drying the fingertips before applying the neutral liquid polish.

Step-by-step pedicure

- Remove old nail polish from the nails of both the feet.
- File nails of the left foot with emery board. Shape the nails straight across. Do not cut or file the corners of the nails. Smooth rough edges of the nails with the fine side of emery board.
- Repeat the above procedure on right foot.
- Place left foot in warm soapy water, followed by the right foot. Dry both the feet and apply cuticle solution with a cotton-tipped orangewood stick under the free edge of each toenail.
- Massage each toe with cuticle cream or oil.

Foot massage

- Apply cocount oil or cream all over the feet.
- Commence the massage with fingers, with firm rotating movements beginning from the instep down to the centre of the toes.
- Slide the thumbs firmly back to instep and repeat the same movement.
- Slide the thumbs back to the hollow of the heel, then back to the base of the foot and repeat the same movement.
- Start at the heel and work down to the centre of the toes.

- Slide back forcefully towards the heel and repeat the same movement up each side of the foot.
- Hold the small toe in one hand and the big toe in the other hand. Give three rotating movements. Repeat the same operation with the other toes.
- Slide your right hand to the ankle and the palm of your left hand to the ball of the foot. Apply six rotating movements.
- Take over the right foot and repeat the same steps.
- Take off the coconut oil from both the feet with a warm moist towel.
- Apply witchhazel or astringent with a cotton pledget to the feet.
- Complete with dusting powder.

Leg massage

Extend the foot massage to and over the knee. A leg massage not only beautifies and strengthens the skin of your leg but at the same time, it is a big relief after a hectic day because it relaxes and rejuvenates all your lcg muscles and bones.

Superfluous hair on the face and body

Superfluous hair on the face and body is one of the most embarrassing beauty problems. There can be many reasons for this unwanted hair growth known as **hirsutism**, such as congenital causes, hormone imbalance, pregnancy, irregular menstruation, menopause, mental tension, prolonged illness, worries and shock. Most of the women suffering from excessive growth of unwanted hair are in the age group of 15 to 25 years. Electrolysis is the only permanent treatment for removal of the facial hair.

- *Unwanted hair on the face*: They usually grow on the chin, above the upper lip and on the forehead.
- *Under-arm hair:* Shaving is the quickest process for getting rid of under-arm hair. You may use depilatory cream, which gives a smooth finish. Waxing over this area is a painful process.
- *Arms and legs hair*: Do not shave over this area. Waxing or applying depilatory cream is convenient.
- *Thigh hair*: Shaving is not recommended. Use depilatory cream with care. The soft skin may become blotchy. It may cause redness, which will subside in three to four days.
- *Breast hair*: Electrolysis is suggested to remove hair on the breasts. Avoid plucking or use of razor.
- *Stomach hair*: Electrolysis is recommended. It gives tiny scabs, which take some time to heal. Avoid plucking, shaving or depilatory creams.

Use of chemical depilatories

Chemical depilatories are generally available as a cream, paste, or powder mixed with water into a paste. These are mainly used for the removal of unwanted hair from the legs. A skin test is necessary before use of these chemical depilatories to ascertain if the skin is sensitive to the action of the depilatory. To do this test, select a hairless part of the arm, apply a little of the cream depilatory and leave it on the skin for 5 to 10 minutes. If there is no sign of redness or swelling, the depilatory can be used with safety over a large area of the skin. The following procedure is employed for the use of any depilatory paste or powder:

- The powder is mixed to form a smooth paste.
- After the skin has been cleansed and dried, a thick layer of the depilatory cream is applied over the part to be treated.
- The surrounding skin is protected with vaseline.
- Depending on the thickness of the hair, the depilatory is retained for five to ten minutes.
- The depilatory and the hair are then washed off with warm water.
- Finally, pat the skin dry and apply a little cold cream.

How to prepare wax yourself

Collect the following ingredients:

- Eight parts sugar syrup
- One part lemon juice
- One part mustard oil
- Two parts of water

Mix the above ingredients on medium heat for 45 minutes. When the mixture turns brown in colour, remove it from the heat and add a little glycerine to it. Let it get cold. Honey can also be used to make hot wax. Add five spoonfuls of honey instead of sugar syrup, in case of a hot wax, especially.

Procedure for applying hot and cold waxing

Waxing may be applied to remove the superfluous hair over the face and body, at cheeks, chin, upper lip, nape area, arms and legs. The following general procedure is employed:

- Remove clothes from the part to be treated and sit or seat the customer in a comfortable position.
- Wash the skin with a mild soap and water. Rinse thoroughly and dry.
- Spread talcum powder over the skin surface.
- Melt wax over the stove and test the temperature and consistency of the heated wax, applying a little over the arm, leg or area to be treated.
- Spread warm wax evenly over the skin surface with a spatula or fingertips, following the same direction as the hair growth.

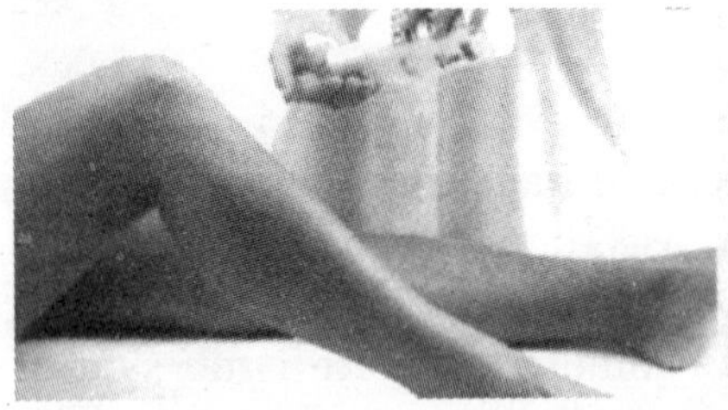
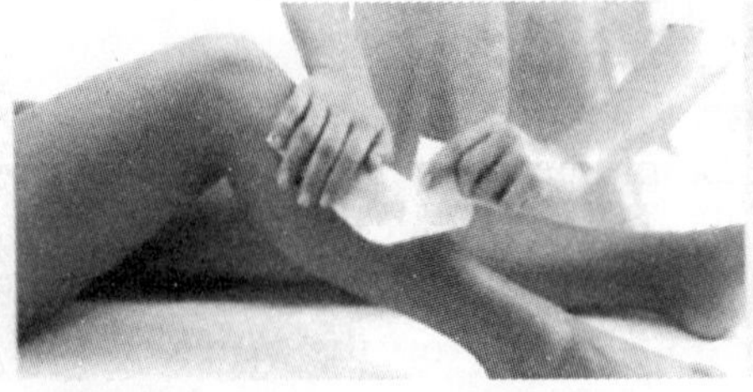
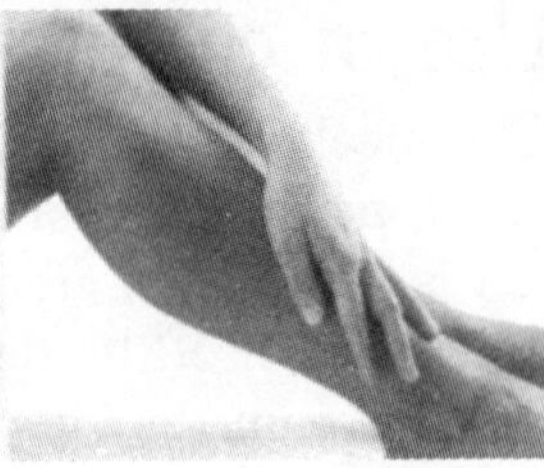

- Allow the wax to cool and harden.
- Quickly pull off the adhering wax against the direction of the hair growth.
- Dust off the remaining powder from skin.
- Apply an emollient cream or an antiseptic lotion to the area treated.

  Warning: Do not use a wax depilatory under the arms, over warts and moles, abrasions or irritated or inflamed skin.

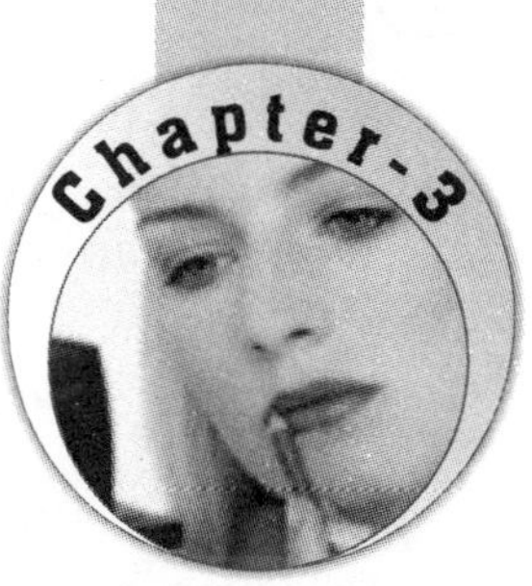

Beauty Tips

A very famous writer once said—"A woman is as old as she looks." Women have been obsessed with their looks since times immemorial. Various techniques and products were used to maintain the beauty of face and body. Today, in the modern age, women are even more aware of the necessity to enhance and maintain their beauty. A good skin, cleanliness and pampering of the body helps in staying beautiful for a longer time. Facials and treatments are also beneficial. Make-up applied in the right manner does wonders for even a plain looking woman. The following tips will surely prove useful.

How to apply make-up

Role of foundation

Foundation cream or lotion plays an important role in giving a smooth look to the face. It is applied on the facial skin as a base of make-up so as to heighten the glow on the skin. The correct use of foundation makes your face attractive. Foundation is applied before make-up. First clean your face with deep cleansing milk. Foundation is not only the base of make-up, it is also the protecting agent of the skin as well as an effective medium to hide pimples, shadows and other spots. If you have a dry skin, choose lanolin mixed foundation cream. For oily skin, cake foundation is good. Apply foundation according to the shape and structure of your face as explained below:

Shape of your face	***Application of foundation***
Round face	Use a dark shade of foundation.
Square face	Use a dark shade of foundation over the jaw and chin.
Diamond-shaped face	Use a dark shade of foundation.
Black spots under eyes	Hide under a coating of light foundation.
Broad nose	Apply a dark shade on each side of the nose, to make it look thinner.
Double chin	Apply dark foundation on its underneath part.
Raised cheek-bone	Apply dark shade foundation below the cheek-bone.

How to apply foundation

- Shake the foundation to make sure the ingredients are evenly blended.
- Take a small quantity in the left palm and apply on the face with fingers of the right hand.
- Dot a little foundation over forehead, nose, cheek, chin and neck (otherwise the neck will appear darker than the face).

- Foundation is applied with an upward motion from the chin onwards with fingertips.
- If the skin is too dry, apply glycerine with a cotton swab before applying foundation.
- If your skin is too oily, use astringent lotion mixed with a few drops of rose water or lemon juice.
- Cleanse your eyebrows and eyelashes to remove any extra foundation sticking on them.
- In case of blemishes on the skin, hide with an extra dabbing of foundation.

How to apply cream

Often, women apply cream on their face in large quantity without realising that they are simply wasting it. Cream keeps the skin beautiful and healthy. It covers the skin with its oily film preventing the cells from developing dryness. Before applying cream, clean your face with the cleanser to remove dirt from the skin and open its pores.

- To apply cream correctly, take it on your fingers, apply it and massage slowly upwards to the middle portion of your face.
- Now apply the cream on the middle of the forehead and massage from the inward corners of the eyebrows and outwards.
- Now apply cream on the upper lip and move towards the cheeks.
- Apply cream below the lower lip and move down till you reach below the chin.

How to apply powder

Powder is an effective beauty aid to make the skin look soft and attractive. It is available in two forms: cake and powder. Choose a shade which goes with your skin, otherwise the skin of your face will look blotchy. Do not forget to use powder on your neck. Dust off extra powder with a cotton wool pad.

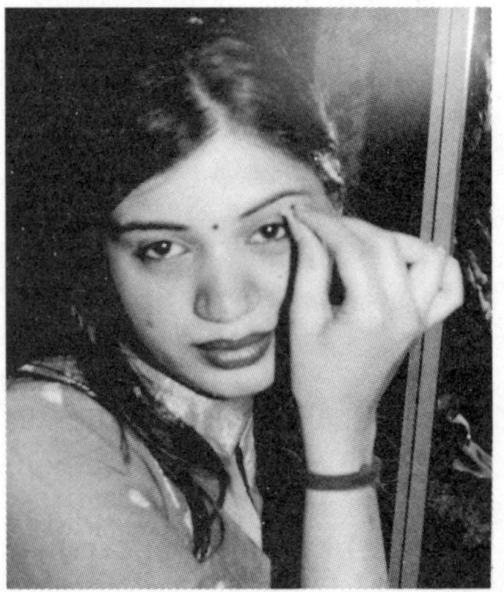

How to make the eyes beautiful

Applying foundation, eye shadow, mascara, eyebrow pencil and eyeliner are various steps for making your eyes beautiful. Make sure that the foundation covers the eyelids completely, then powder over this to give a matt surface to work on.

- Apply the eyelid shadow first in light strokes, then crease shadow and finally apply shadow on the brow bone. Eye shadow is used on eyelids between eyebrow and eyelashes and applied with fingers.

- Now apply mascara very carefully, in upward strokes on top lashes and in downward strokes on the bottom ones. Apply one coat, allow it to dry, then apply a second coat. For a thick, soft look without fibres, powder between each coat. Finally, separate the lashes with a dry brush for a natural, feathery look.
- Apply the eyebrow pencil lightly to give a natural curve to the brows. Tweeze away any hair, which spoil the line, but below the brow only.
- Now apply an eyeliner. Choose a shadow which is close to that of the shadow on your lid and make a soft, smudgy line, not a hard one.

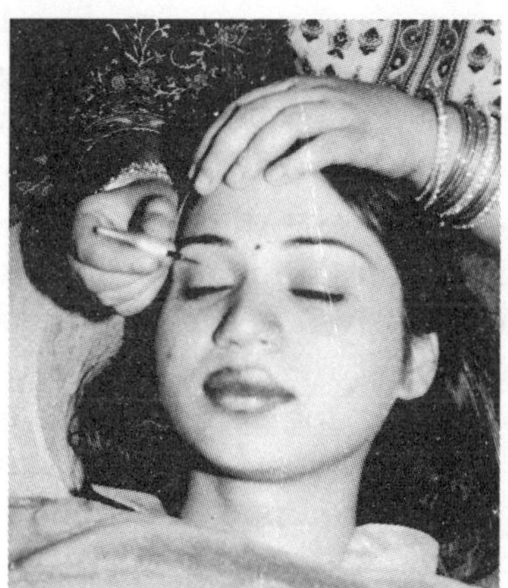

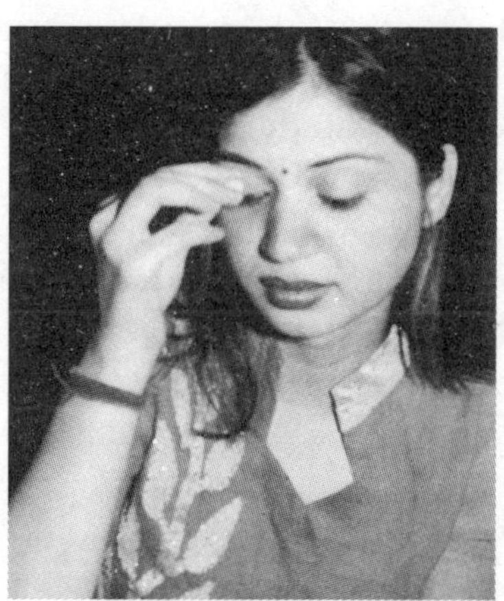

- Eyes can be made to appear larger or smaller through the use of eye shadow. Round eyes can be made to look longer by extending the eye shadow beyond the outer corner of the eyes. Small eyes can be made to appear larger by extending the shadow slightly above, beyond and below the eyes. For deep sunken eyes, use very little shadow on lids, nearest the temples and leave untouched the part next to the nose and inner corners of the eyes.

How to apply lip colour

- Examine the texture of your lips. If they are hard, soften with lip balm or moisturiser.
- Apply a thin film of creamy foundation over the whole of the lip area and powder lightly.
- First draw in the outline of your lips with a well-filled brush.
- Now fill in the colour very carefully. Two colours used separately or blended give a good result.
- If lip colours tend to smudge into the surrounding skin, blot with a tissue and re-apply.
- Apply clear or toning lip gloss for a shiny look.

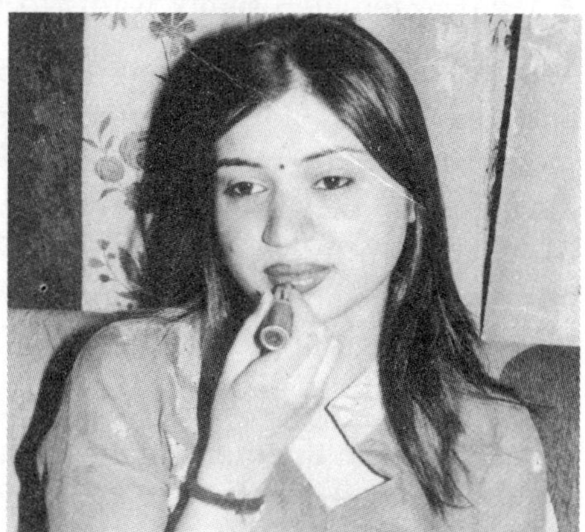

Beauty tips for your baby

A little everyday care ensures that the natural beauty of your baby does not fade away too soon. Here are a few basic guidelines to a beauty regime for your kids. It is best to ensure that the rosy cheeks, pearly teeth and the shining hair stay for long. Little ones need a personal care routine as much an adults do.

Little babies are blessed with soft and silky skin. Nourish your baby's skin with a regular oil massage before the bath. After the bath, use a light moisturising lotion. In hot weather, massage reacts adversely and produces rashes or itching. If this happens, stop all products immediately. During the summer season, use powder on clean, dry skin. Remember, the sun's harmful rays may cause the delicate skin to burn and peel. Bathe your baby twice a day using a glycerine soap during summer. Avoid using soap on the face. It is too harsh and causes drying of the skin. Clean your baby's face with a non-soap based face wash.

It is preferable to oil your baby's hair once a week to keep it shining and prevent split ends. Do not use too much oil. Apply a good conditioner on the hair but not on the scalp. The conditioner flattens down the cells of the hair and gives it smoothness, shine and easy manageability. A haircut once in six weeks is a must. Do not forget to wash the hair whenever it gets dirty, even if it means doing it everyday. Use a mild shampoo and condition the hair each time. Wet hair is extremely weak and breaks easily, so use a wide toothed comb to untangle the hair. Never use a brush on wet hair. Allow the hair to dry naturally as a hair dryer tends to dry out the hair, and the hair gets brittle. If the hair is long, keep it loosely tied during the night to prevent it from getting knotted. Always use mild products which contain herbal ingredients.

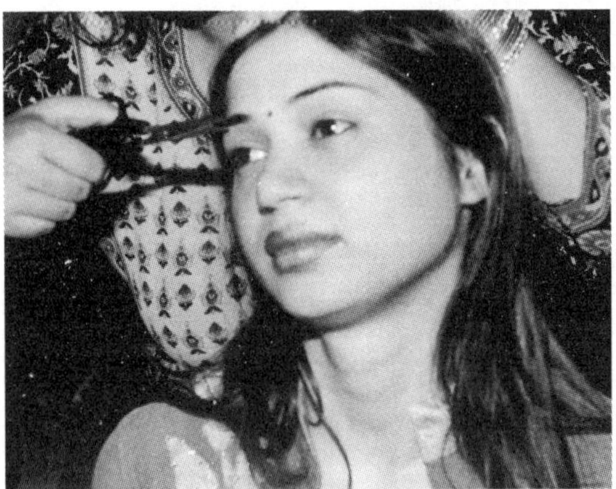

Beauty tips during periods

A teenage female usually wants to know what **menses** is.

Menstruation is the monthly discharge of blood and mucous along with broken down cells and tissue bits of the uterus. Menses commences at age of 12–13 years and stops at menopause in a female when she reaches the age of 45 or 50. The periods stop temporarily during pregnancy, the first few months following delivery and sometimes, though rarely, in many women in lactation period. The length of each cycle could vary a few days from the normal of 28 days. Sometimes, there is a deviation in the amount of blood lost, number of bleeding days, duration of bleeding-free period in case of disorders of the uterus or functioning of hormonal imbalance.

The changes in the menstrual cycle usually happen due to the female sex hormones from the regulating centre—the pituitary gland influenced by the brain. The pituitary hormone stimulates the ovaries to secrete estrogen. The ovaries begin the secretion of progesterone which makes the endometrium spongy in preparation for the fertilised egg to get settled in the uterus. In the absence of fertilisation, 14 days from the ovulation, there is a sudden drop in the level of progesterone and estrogen, the inner lining of the uterus starts breaking up and passes out mixed with blood as menstrual flow. In few cases, periods occur in the first couple of months of pregnancy due to a lower level of pregnancy hormones in the blood. Most women find discomfort in menses due to pelvic congestion or an infection. The main disorders of menstruation are absence of periods (Amenorrhoea), scanty and painful discharge (Dysmenorrhoea), profuse bleeding (Menorrhagia) and irregular menstruation (Metrorrhagia).

Problems during periods

Pigmentation of the skin is a major problem during periods. What we want is an even toned, translucent, radiant and blemish-free skin during these days. The melanin in the skin is the culprit. The amount and distribution of this pigment determines the skin colour and the difference in the colour of the skin. The imbalance in both types can stay on just the upper layer of the skin or run deep as well. If spots or discolouration run deep, they usually appear bluish.

Hyperpigmentation is usually faced by women during periods. The common problems related to pigmentation are **Melasma**: A brownish discolouration that usually starts after pregnancy but tends to persist (usually seen on cheeks, forehead and nose) and these increase in pigmentation before and during menstruation. There are several ointments available in the market to cope with pigmentation. Home-made remedies like cucumber, milk cream, turmeric powder, gram flour (*besan*) and fuller's earth (*multani mitti*) also work well to get rid of pigmentation during periods or pregnancy. Ointments and home-made remedies can cause allergic reactions and dryness of the skin in some women.

Treating yourself to a facial just before periods is beneficial, because it can help to clear away the dead skin that produces an extra oily complexion and blocks the pores of the skin. A facial after the periods is equally beneficial as it helps to refine the skin's texture. A rest is must after the facial. After you have had blackheads extracted, you will be looking a bit blotchy. Don't bother to wash or style your hair before a facial. Facial brings out toxins and the skin looks best for about a week after a facial.

During periods, skin cleansing, moisturising and application of face pack are essential routines that help the skin to retain its glowing radiance. They play an important role in maintaining the skin soft and smooth. Use yoghurt and lemon cleansing milk for oily skin during the menstruation period to clear the clogged skin.

To prepare home-made cleansing milk: Mix one teaspoon each of yoghurt and lemon juice and apply on the face. When dry, wipe it away with a cotton pad. In case the skin is dry, almond cleansing milk benefits. To prepare it, collect the following ingredients:

Almond Oil	:	1 tsp (teaspoon)
Powdered Almond	:	4-5
Warm Milk	:	1 tbsp (tablespoon)

Mix all the above ingredients and apply on the face. When dry, wipe it away with a cotton pad.

You may prepare a moisturiser with natural ingredients yourself. Collect the following ingredients :

Almond Oil	:	½ tsp
Honey	:	¼ tsp
Pulp of Peach or Banana	:	1 tsp
Olive Oil	:	¼ tsp
Apple Juice	:	1 tsp
Milk	:	1 tsp

Mix all the above ingredients, apply it on the face and massage the skin gently every night to prevent dryness and keep it wrinkle-free.

Here is a face pack for refreshing and relaxing during periods. Mix the following ingredients to prepare this pack and apply on your face:

Egg Yolk	:	One egg
Honey	:	½ tsp
Almond Oil	:	1 tsp
Curd	:	1tsp
Oatmeal	:	½ tsp
Mashed Banana	:	1 tsp

Fragrant, soothing and sacred sandalwood is a good antiseptic to stimulate the immune system. It helps ward off infection, relieves inflammation, soothes dry itchy skin and leaves a calming and cooling effect. Honey mixed with sandalwood powder leaves a moisturising effect, rejuvenates all types of skin and cures acne and rashes on the skin.

Beauty tips for the pregnant

Pregnancy can change your appearance due to rapid hormonal changes, which cause dry, flaky skin or a blotchy acne-prone complexion. The body undergoes many changes when pregnant. Skin is the first thing to bear the brunt of it. Some of the common problems include very dry, itchy skin, melasma, acne and stretch marks. Do not despair, these can be treated during and after pregnancy. Usually, from the second trimester of pregnancy, a pregnant woman might suddenly find herself with very dry, taut skin that is sand papery to the touch, especially around the stomach, hands and legs. Do not be alarmed, generally the condition vanishes after delivery. But till then, be sure to keep your skin extra moisturised with a creamy body lotion. Almond oil or cocoa butter based creams tend to work wonders in soothing the skin during this period when applied after bath.

Melasma (pregnancy mask)

Melasma is basically brown pigmentation around the eyes, on the cheeks and above the lip. The hormonal changes combined with exposure to the sun can cause this complexion problem. To avoid this, wear a broad spectrum sunscreen that blocks the ultra-violet rays. Avoid laser treatment, as it tends to worsen the condition rather than rectify it.

Stretch marks and acne

For most women, the skin tends to clear up during pregnancy due to extra blood flow in the system. Stretch marks are undoubtedly the biggest problems that almost all pregnant women worry about. This happens when the skin loses its elasticity due to the stretching of the upper and lower layers of the skin. They generally appear as red marks which form white stripe-like marks across the stomach. With timely treatment with vitamin E oil, the stretch marks may lighten. Some of the pregnant women experience hair loss, dry or excessively oily scalps. A regular hair care and balanced diet, however, improves conditions. Have a weekly massage to take care of your split ends.

The first three months

A woman can have a radiant serenity when she is pregnant. But pregnancy can also be a time of difficulty for a mother-to-be. There are additional physical strains to cope with and there can be mental ones, too. Friends and relatives may give confusing and conflicting advice. In the midst of such pressures, a pregnant woman often has no room for her beauty care. But it is very important for an expectant mother to spend some of her time thinking about herself. If the expectant mother is relaxed and healthy, then her baby stands a good chance of being healthy too. The 40 weeks of pregnancy have several beauty problems as well as some beauty bonuses. Nature may prove very good to some mothers-to-be. They may find that pregnancy has produced unexpected benefits like clear skin, glowing cheeks and glossy hair. An expectant mother may become beautiful, if she starts taking extra beauty care from the very beginning.

During the first trimester of pregnancy, there is a great hormonal activity in the body, which aggravates acne, lifeless hair and lack of energy. The figure becomes plump and lumpy. The joy of realising that you are going to be mother may be clouded by doubts and disappointment over the way you look disfigured. Start by thinking positive about your beauty care and a daily beauty routine, which will have a tremendous effect upon your looks and morale. Spots appearing on your face, chest or back should not worry you as the increased hormonal activity in your body is causing this temporary upset. Clean skin thoroughly in the morning and evening, treat spotty areas with astringent and a medicated skin lotion. Disguise the ones on your face with a camouflage stick, followed by a light make-up. Never squeeze any spot anywhere to get rid of it, for it may leave a permanent scar.

When you are pregnant, pay special attention to lubricate the skin on your stomach, buttocks and breasts. Apply plenty of skin conditioning cream after your bath and rub a little baby oil or olive oil every night. Stretch marks are very difficult to remove after the birth, but lubrication of skin at this time can prevent them altogether. Keep lubricating throughout the nine months of pregnancy period.

You need more nutrients, not more calories. Cut out fried, sweet, stodgy and fatty foods. Fish provides vitamin D which you need at this stage. Drink a glass of milk in a day, it fulfils the need of calcium. Morning sickness can be avoided by eating digestive biscuits. Take smaller meals more frequently during the day.

Get as much fresh air as you can. Avoid really strenuous exercise during the crucial first three months. Go to bed early. The most radiant mother-to-be of all is the rested one.

The second trimester

Beauty care taken early in pregnancy now begins to pay dividends. Most mothers find that nausea stops being a serious problem by the fourth month, and hair and skin conditions improve at this stage. If you have watched your diet in the initial months, your bump will be a manageable size. Cleanse and tone skin twice a day. Apply moisturiser under the make-up. If the cheeks are too rosy, tone them down with a grey-tinged face powder over matt beige foundation. Avoid over doing the toning down. Keep the make-up simple .

Continue with daily stomach, bottom and breast lubrication and pay special attention to skin freshness. Underarm depilation and deodorising is essential. Make bath time relaxing and enjoyable and follow every bath with a light foot massage to soften the skin and stimulate blood circulation. Night cramps are often a problem at this stage.

Keep a strict watch on your diet and weight gain. Total weight gain during pregnancy should be about 12 kgs. Remember, **toxaemia** (blood poisoning) and **high blood pressure** are dangers for overweight mothers-to-be and so are **varicose veins.**

Keep walking with your doctor's advice. Wear comfortable shoes and walk slowly. It is important to keep up light exercise as per your doctor's approval. Going to bed early is a good habit during this period. The most comfortable position in bed is lying on your side with one leg slightly in front of the other, one hand under the pillow and the other by your side. That way the weight is evenly distributed.

The final months

This is the time for organisation and final preparations to welcome the baby. Take good care of yourself too, you will need a lot of energy in the coming months. Dryness and blotchiness are sometimes problems at the end of the pregnancy period. Take care to nourish your skin properly. Use a covering foundation during the day. If your face looks fat, use shading to disguise the chubbiness. Give your body plenty of skin cream in the last two months. If you intend to breastfeed your baby, keep your nipples soft with a special cream to help prevent cracking.

Increase milk and high protein food in your diet. Keep your iron intake high, too. Drink fresh orange juice instead of tea or coffee. A high vitamin C intake helps protect you against infections. When labour begins, have a good meal. You will need all your strength and you may not get another meal for many hours. A good sleep is a necessity during the final month. If you find it difficult to get to sleep, have a warm glass of milk the last thing at night or relax in a warm bath just before bedtime.

Have your hair trimmed and set this month. You will be far too busy next month to go to a hairdresser. Your hair may become a bit greasy this month, so freshen it between the shampoos by putting a piece of cheese cloth or muslin over the bristles of your brush and press them through it. Much of the dirt and grease will be caught over the cloth.

Post-natal care of your beauty

Having a baby takes a great deal of energy. Even though you have been following a good ante-natal beauty programme, you are bound to feel tired and exhausted for the first few months after the birth of the child. Your skin may be looking dull and your hair lacking in shine.

Make sure that your diet is rich in nutrients, e.g., plenty of vitamin C, proteins and minerals. Keep up the iron supplement you took before your baby was born. If your skin looks pale and sallow, use a pink-tinged make-up for a month or so to give you colour and add a little blusher. Put on light eye make-up and lipstick everyday. Choose bright and pretty colours.

Your hair needs special care. Have it trimmed regularly and wash it frequently. Use a conditioner after each shampoo. Watch your nails to prevent cracking and splitting. Be lavish with perfume.

Beauty tips in 20s

In 20s, the metabolic rate is high enough to ensure that a low-fat eating plan coupled with regular exercise will result in an attractive body for you. You will have high hormone levels to ensure gain in muscle mass. Perform regular weight-bearing exercise. But excessive exercising and dieting can lead to a drop in estrogen. Best bets for fat burning include aerobic exercises, such as cycling, jogging, speed walking and hip-hop dancing. An inactive person will start to lose muscle mass and unused energy will be stored in the form of fat—not only around hips and thighs, but around the internal organs too.

Avoid fried food, it's bad for the skin. Coconut water or juice will help. I always suggest a light make-up at this age, which provides handsome dividends in 30s and 40s. Your skin glows in 20s and has an even texture. Some people develop adult acne. Develop a good cleansing regimen and stick to sunscreen. The muscle strength is at its peak and the lungs are at their maximum aerobic capacity needing 1200 mgs of calcium a day to build bone density.

Beauty tips in 30s

You will observe several changes in your body in 30s. Overall muscle strength drops. Bone mass declines at the rate of one percent a year and one becomes fragile. The ratio of bony fat to the muscle increases causing extra flab and the cholesterol continues to rise, increasing the risk of heart attack.

Proper care to nourish the body should be taken to maintain the muscle and bone density and also to keep the fat level down. Make sure that your diet is good but fat-free. It is seen that wrong eating habits lead to anaemia, hyperacidity and bowel problems. A sedentary lifestyle leads to the onset of obesity, back and joint problems, hypertension, low backache, spondylitis, respiratory problems, diabetes, varicose veins and even heart diseases. The following eating habits are suggested:

- Eat until you are 80% satisfied.
- Eat fresh food: either steamed, stir-fried or poached.
- If you are non-vegetarian, eat lots of fish and small quantities of meat occasionally.
- Avoid alcohol. It is observed that the consumption of alcohol by the female sex leads to breast cancer and other fatal diseases.
- Drink a lot of water, at least six to eight glasses of water a day.
- Don't forget your daily calcium consumption prescribed, i.e., 1200 mgs. per day. Calcium is important to help ward off osteoporosis. Consume low fat dairy products and leafy green vegetables to supplement the calcium demand of the body.
- Choose whole-wheat *chapatis*, bread, cereals and unpolished rice.
- Opt for low-fat milk, yoghurt, cheese and *paneer*.
- At this age fats, oils, sugar, desserts and pastries are dangerous.
- Decrease the consumption of salt in your diet.
- Avoid eating too much of red meat, milk, eggs, fried foods and sweets.
- Increase the intake of whole grain cereals, legumes, sprouts and buttermilk.
- Have a regular exercise plan—be it a walk, a musical dancing, swimming, exercise bike, treadmill, brisk walking, Yoga or aerobics.

Fine lines begin to develop around your eyes and mouth. Skin pores increase in size and the hair begins to lose volume. Start using an eye cream to hide the fine lines and dark circles under the eyes. Use moisturiser with an SPF factor and condition your hair.

Beauty tips in 40s

Human body is like a machine, if you leave it out it starts rusting. Obesity is common at this age, especially among those who had neglected their body in 30s. Height reduction begins at 40s as your skeletal structure starts to weaken, the muscles, ligaments and tendons tend to lose flexibility, extra weight on the bottom and thighs looks irritating as a part of the ageing process. Oil production continues to decrease, wrinkles and spots become more obvious as collagen levels decrease and the skin starts losing its elasticity. The skin appears dull and less smooth due to the dead skin build up, furrow and expression lines deepen. Grey hairs increase, white blood cells become a common problem in the body and sexual dysfunction sets in after the age of 40.

Thyroid and eyesight, diabetes and hypertension, breasts losing their firmness, wrinkles and stretch marks on the face are common disorders in 40s. Estrogen levels begin to drop, making it easier for fat to accumulate around the stomach and waist when the skeletal structure starts weakening. Menopause itself brings along various problems. The female hormone or estrogen is manufactured in the body as long as the monthly cycle continues. It helps in maintaining strong bones and keeps the skin supple.

To maintain the strength of the bones, a regular stretching exercise routine and intake of calcium is essential in 40s. They help fight the ageing process by building the bone mass. Aerobic exercises keep fat at bay and the muscles intact. To keep the skin and hair healthy, use a nourishing cream, non-clogging moisturiser and hair conditioner.

Beauty tips in 50s

Lot of changes develop among women in 50s. After menopause, the bone mass in the body further drops, weight piles up, skin becomes dry and itchy, double chin appears, neck gets looser and less elastic, pores become smaller, wrinkles become more obvious, brown spots and scaly patches develop on the face, neck and the body.

Continue with a good cleansing and moisturising routine. Wrong eating habits and lack of exercise harm the body. A light exercise and regular practice of Yoga are good ways to remain fit and healthy.

Tips to conceal blemishes

Concealers are a fast and effective way to disguise blemishes, so that your skin looks perfect. Apply concealers after applying foundation and this is the best technique to conceal blemishes. They are applied only to specific areas and would be disturbed if the foundation is applied over the top. Concealers are of several types such as stick, cream and liquid.

- **Stick Concealers:** These are easy to apply and you can simply stroke them straight on the skin.
- **Cream Concealers:** These usually come in a tube and are applied with a sponge-tipped applicator and give a very natural finish effect. However, the coverage is not as thick as in case of a stick type.
- **Liquid Concealers:** These come in a tube. Just squeeze a tiny amount of product onto your finger and smooth over the affected area. This is a cream-to-powder formulation which sticks on like a cream and dries to a velvety powder finish.

When choosing a concealer, look for the colour nearest to your own skin tone rather than a lighter one. Covering the problem area with a paler shade will accentuate it.

If you have spots and blemishes

Use a medicated stick concealer as it contains ingredients to deal with pimples or blemishes as well as cover it. Apply the concealer on the acne or the pimple or the blemish, and then smooth away the edges with a clean cotton bud.

In case of under-eye shadows

Hide under-eye shadows with a few drops of concealer. Apply the concealer directly onto the clean skin, then apply powder or an all-in-one foundation on the top. Use your ring finger to blend, not to drag at the delicate skin.

Tips to beautify a warm skin (delicate skin)

Opt for tawny neutral shades of make-up applied with a light touch to enhance your basic colouring. A warm skin comprises a dark blonde hair, brown, blue, hazel or green eyes and a warm skin tone.

- After applying a light, tinted moisturiser, stroke the concealer onto problem areas. Apply the concealer with a cotton bud in case of thread veins or spots on the skin.
- Dip a powder puff into the loose powder and lightly apply on the face. This will absorb the excess oil and leave your skin beautifully matt. Dust off the excess powder.
- Sweep peach eyeshadow over your entire eyelid and then blend with your natural skin tone.
- Use an eyeshadow brush to work a small amount of soft brown eyeshadow into the crease of your eyelids, sweeping it out towards the outer corners of your eyes. Work a little underneath your lower lashes too. Finish with two coats of brown or black mascara.
- Apply a light shade of lipstick.
- Apply blusher covering your cheeks, forehead and chin.

Tips to beautify a cool skin (pale skin)

Pale-skinned women look fabulous with strong, cool shades of cosmetics. This look suits you if you have a medium to dark brown hair, you have a cool (China Doll) skin tone and your eyes are brown, blue, grey or green.

- Apply a foundation or tinted moisturiser. Blend in a few dots of blusher. Dust with loose powder.
- Smudge a cool ivory shadow over your eyelids, right up to your eyebrows. Blend it with a cotton swab. Use an eyeshadow on your eyelids to emphasise the colour of your eyes.
- Now move on to your eyelashes and apply two thin coats of black mascara.
- Slick your eyebrows into place with an eyebrow brush.
- Choose a clear shade of berry lipstick.

Tips for five-minute quick make-up

When you do not have much time to spare, try this quick routine face make-up to give a simple sexy look:

- The all-in-one foundation powder formulation gives your skin the medium coverage (One minute).
- Apply cream eyeshadow straight from the stick, which is easy to apply. Opt for brown shade as it brings out the colour of your eyes and gives them a sexy, sultry finish (Half a minute).
- Blend in your eyeshadow to brush over the top with translucent loose powder. This will tone down the colour (One minute).
- Apply a coat of mascara to your lower lashes as well as the upper one (One minute).
- A warm berry red blusher will give your skin a fabulous flush. Apply it with a blusher brush, sweeping it from your cheeks up towards your eyes (Half a minute).
- Choose a berry shade of lipstick to add instant bold colour to your lips. Cover your lower lip first then apply on your upper lip (Half a minute).

Tips for a classic make-up

A classic make-up always makes a pleasing impact on all types of faces, irrespective of the age and complexion.

- Apply a sheer all-in-one foundation powder to give your skin the perfect coverage.
- Use eyelash colours for eye make-up to give your eyes a fresh look.
- Apply a pale ivory eyeshadow across your entire eyelid using a blender brush. Apply two thin coats of brown-black mascara.
- Lightly fill in any gaps with a toning eyeshadow for a soft, natural effect.
- Your lips are the focus of your look. Use a toning red lip pencil. Rest your elbow on a hard surface while you outline your lips, to prevent wobbling.
- Use a lip brush to fill in with a bold shade of red lipstick. Apply a coat, blot with tissue, then reapply for a long lasting finish.

Tips for summer make-up having freckles

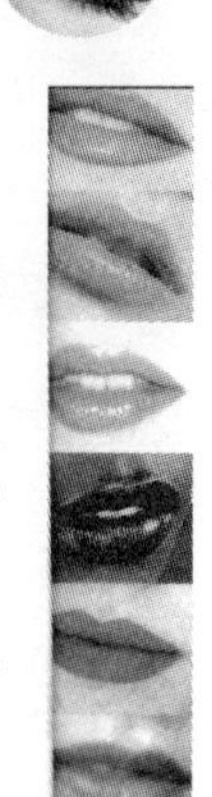

If you want a fresh look for your skin having freckles, the following make-up routine is suggested:

- Avoid heavy make-up and heavy foundations during summer. However, tinted moisturiser is the perfect solution as it both nourishes your skin and lightly covers any minor blemishes.
- If you have freckles, don't try to hide them. Use a mid-brown eyebrow pencil and dot the freckles on the nose and cheeks.
- Dust your skin with loose powder over your temples.

- Apply eyeshadow, blend it with a brush over your eyelids.
- Keep the mascara to a minimum. Choose a natural-looking brown or brown/black shade. In summer, a waterproof type should be used, but remember, you will need a waterproof eye make-up remover, too.
- Don't overpower the look with bold lipstick. Opt for a muted brown-pink shade, close to your natural lip colour or use a tinted lip gloss for a natural sheen.

Tips for make-up to look younger

Wearing out of fashion make-up adds years to your appearance. A dull, lifeless skin-tone can make you look aged. There are now foundations and concealers in the market especially designed to deal with this problem. These bounce the light away from your skin and give an illusion of added vitality and help disguise the problem areas with fine lines, under-eye shadows, blemishes and wrinkles.

Apply foundation with a damp sponge, blending away harsh edges. Apply a concealer, dotting it on to the under-eye shadows, blemishes and thread veins with a brush. Apply a little at a time and blend it thoroughly. Avoid the extremes of fashion and bright colours when you are over 40. Forget about adding colour to your skin with foundation. The cream variety of blusher is a good bet to provide your skin a soft glow. Dot the blusher on to your skin and blend with your fingertips. Lightly set your foundation and blusher with translucent powder. Applying too much powder can make it settle into fine lines and wrinkles on the face. So aim for a light touch which will just blot out shine and set your make-up. The best way to apply powder is only to blot the area that needs it, then brush away the excess, stroking the brush downwards to prevent tiny layers on the skin.

Apply a cream-to-powder eye shadow, which dries quickly to a super-soft powder finish. Give eyeliners a miss. Harsh lines of colour close to your eyes can be hard and unflattering. Smudge a little neutral-toned powder eyeshadow under your lower lashes with a clean cotton bud.

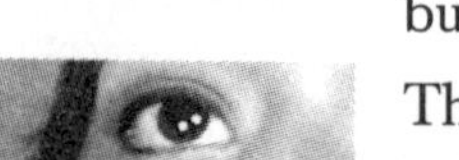

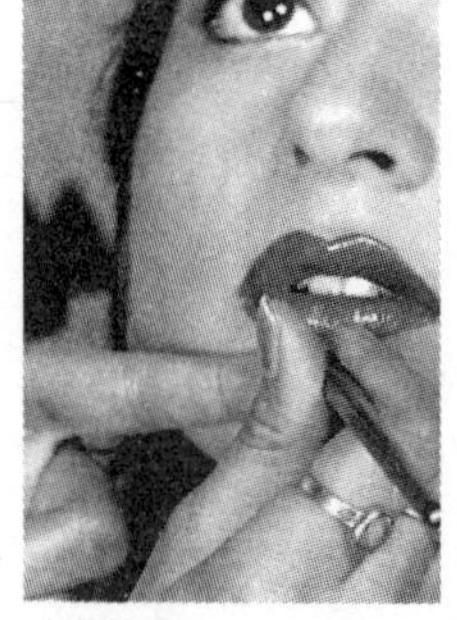

The complexion fades slightly over the years. The black mascara you wear can now look too obvious and harsh. So try switching to a lighter shade for a more flattering effect. Apply two thin coats. Allow the first to dry thoroughly before you apply the second coat.

If your lip line has started to fade and your lipstick tends to bleed into the lines around your mouth, try using a toning lipliner before you apply lipstick. Outline your upper lip first, then outline your lower lip. Next dust your lips with a loose powder to set the lipliner. Finally, fill in your outline with a moisturising lipstick which gives a glossy shine to your lips.

Aqua make-up (water-proof make-up)

This type of make-up is especially good in summer and rainy season. It does not run when wet. Water-proof products: foundation base, aqua compact, aqua eye colour and lip colour are readily available in the market.

How to apply aqua make-up

- Start with cleansing, toning and moisturising, followed by cold compression after moisturising. Ultra base moisturisers (having water base) are available in the market. It does not give a patchy base in the rainy season. Use Dermacolour to conceal blemishes, dark circles, spots, acne, scars, white patches and tanning.
- Apply pancake for an effective water-proof make-up. The colour of pancake should match with the colour of your skin.
- Use a translucent powder for the make-up base.
- Use cool aqua eye colours for eye make-up in summer. Wet brush with water before using an eyeshadow. Use water-proof eyeliner and aqua mascara for the make-up.
- Apply blusher on cheeks.
- At the end, apply aqua lipstick to colour your lips matching its colour with the colour of the dress you are wearing.

Camouflage cosmetic products

Camouflage products differ from ordinary cosmetics. They have greater covering qualities, are resistant to the harmful rays of the sun and are waterproof. They also have a far greater variety of colours for all ethnic skin tones. Their holding power is better than fashion products and are designed to stay in place when applied. They are also easy to apply and simple to remove. There are five ranges of camouflage products available in single pots for individual use, containing small quantity of all the colours. Dermacolour has a bright orange colour which is useful for applying to hide the dark shadows under the eyes. The orange will take away the blue-black appearance of the shadow without making it look grey.

The basic kit contains the following products:

- Camouflage palettes.
- Cleansing cream, rosewater and witch-hazel for cleansing and removing the grease on the skin.
- Cottonwool, natural sponges, stipple sponges, etc.
- Camouflage powder or unscented talcum powder.
- Cream gauge.

For tiny scars and such other areas, a small brush is more accurate. Small, natural sponges are good for giving a natural effect. The sponge should be made wet to soften it, then squeeze out until it is just damp. Place the required colour in the palm of your hand and press the sponge against the colour to load it. Before using on the facial skin, first apply it on the back of your hand to test the strength of the colour.

How to cover a tattoo

While doing make-up, sometimes you have to cover tattoos. First use a colour on the darkest area of the tattoo which will be hardest to hide. Orange or Veil Rose colour may be applied with a small brush before applying the matching skin shade. Large tattoos are best covered with a natural or tipple sponge in the matching skin tone after the brush work has been completed.

How to cover an indented scar

1. First cover the scar with the shade which matches the surrounding skin tone.
2. Use a colour slightly paler than the matching skin shade. Apply a thin line around the inside edge of the scar with a small brush. Tap it with your fingertip to blend and set in the area.
3. Use a slightly darker cream than the matching skin shade. Apply a thin line around the outside of the scar. Blend it in by tapping lightly with your finger and set in.

How to prepare for make-up

As far as possible, plan everything before starting the make-up, e.g., the shape of your eyes colour, the type of make-up, the colours, base and liner, you will use. Know before you start exactly what the end result will be. For all types of make-up, the basic questions to ask yourself are:

- Why am I using this product?
- Why am I applying it to the area?
- Why have I chosen this colour?
- What will the result look like?

Crystal art

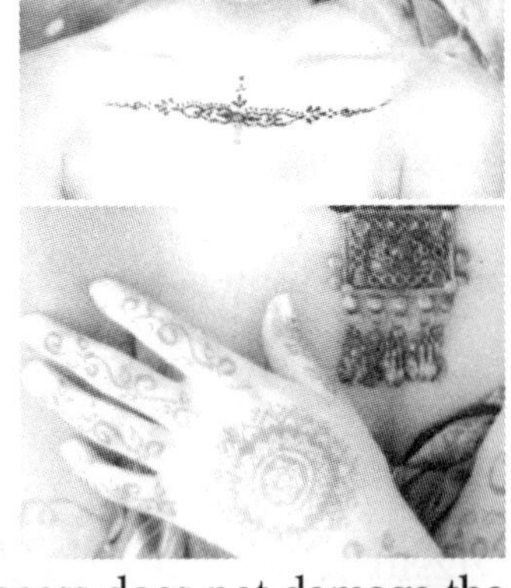

Crystal Art: It is a western style beauty concept which has made it possible to give a new look to the nails, ankles and belly buttons. There is an ancient history of anklets, henna, tattoos and other forms of body embellishments in India. Crystal art placed on your nails, belly button, around the arms or ankles make a unique style on to the human body.

Nail Art: Painting nails and nail art gives a completely new look the nails along with a bit of acrylic nail and some crystals. You can choose an acrylic nail design on the acrylic nail, which lasts longer and this process does not damage the nail. It is not advisable to do nail art on real nails. Nail enamel is first applied on to the nail. Once the polish dries, the chosen design is painted on to the nail polish.The crystals are available in white and other colours and stay for several days when applied.

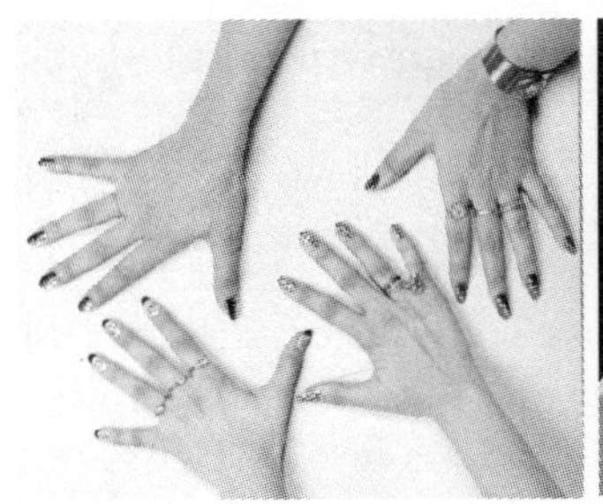

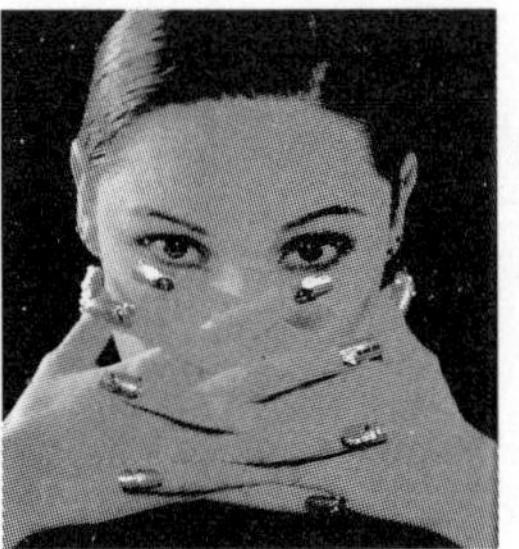

Body tattoos: These are interesting concepts in different designs and colours. The tattoo motifs can be pasted on to the ankles, above the ankle bone or on the back of the shoulder or around the arm. A motif can stay on a place with the help of an adhesive for a few days and can be reused a few times.

Crystal belly jewel: A sexy belly button fixed on your navel or a flat tummy visible on a low-slung sari or a low slung pant and adding the tattoo crystals around it gives a party look.

Be your own beautician on a holiday

When you have a whole day to yourself, i.e., a Sunday or an odd day of a holiday, devote it to beautify yourself. Even in such a short time there are many beauty jobs that you can do and you will end the day looking and feeling relaxed and refreshed. Begin by making sure that you go to bed fairly early the night before your day of beauty. Have a warm bath and a hot drink to make you sleep soundly and start at 8.30 a.m., next morning.

A Day for Beauty

8.30 a.m.: Breakfast. Drink lemon juice of half a lemon in hot, sugarless water.

8.45 a.m.: Limbering exercises in front of an open window, followed by deep breathing. A total relaxation on the floor for one minute.

9.00 a.m.: Lukewarm shower or bath. Dress in jeans and T-shirt or salwar suit and comfortable shoes. Apply moisturiser and a little eye make-up. Do not apply heavy foundation or powder on this day.

9.20 a.m.: Light breakfast. Unsweetened orange juice, 1 boiled egg, crispbread with a scraping of butter, coffee or tea with milk but without sugar.

10.00 a.m.: The next two (2) hours must be devoted to some form of exercise such as swimming, reading or walking. You need to go out in the fresh air, even if it is raining. If you wet your hair in rain, do not bother, re-do your make-up in the afternoon.

12.00 noon: Check that you have all the equipments you need for the afternoon: shampoo, de-fuzzing cream, tweezers for plucking eyebrows, orangestick, nail file, bath oil and lotion, a selection of make-up and other things required, in a tray.

12.30 p.m.: Light lunch. Have raw vegetable salad (grated carrot, shredded cabbage, cauliflower sprigs, chopped celery, watercress, cucumber) with lemon juice dressing. A fresh orange to follow.

1.15 p.m.: Rest for 45 minutes on your bed with your feet slightly higher than your head.

2.00 p.m.: Change into a housecoat and prepare to make your bedroom and bathroom your headquarters for the next three hours. Remove make-up with a cleanser. Take a medium-sized mixing bowl into the bathroom. Stand it on a table and almost fill it with very hot water. Lean your face close to the bowl, having first draped a towel over your head so that the head and the bowl are enclosed in a kind of a towelling tent. Stay in this position so that your face has steam (facial sauna) for few minutes till the bowl remains hot and releases steam. Afterwards, relax for a few minutes to allow your face to cool. Splash with mild astringent. Apply a face pack that suits your skin type. Relax for ten minutes.

2.45 a.m: Remove the face pack with tepid water. Splash the face with astringent again. Apply moisturiser or special treatment cream if your skin is exceptionally dry. Run your bath, pouring in plenty of bath oil or bubble bath.

3.00 p.m.: Relax in bath. Rub your body (apart from your bosom) with a friction mitt to stimulate blood circulation. Relax your skin to get the full benefit of the moisturiser or treatment cream which will penetrate deep into the pores. After your bath, de-fuzz your legs and underarms. Give yourself a full-scale pedicure. Put on your housecoat and underclothes.

3.45 p.m.: Devote the next hour to make-up experiments. Match the colour of your clothes wtih the cosmetics. Look at the clothes you are likely to wear in the next few days and see if any need cleaning, washing or pressing. Pluck your eyebrows, followed by eye make-up. Keep the balance of your face in mind as you do it.

4.45 p.m.: Cleanse your face thoroughly once more. Collect the materials you need to wash and set your hair. Try a conditioner if you have dry, fly-away hair or a lemon rinse for greasy hair. Set your hair.

5.15 p.m.: Dry the hair using a hair-dryer. If you are using a hood hair dryer and your hands are free, give yourself a complete manicure.

6.00 p.m.: After completing the manicure, make-up your face lightly (if you plan to spend the evening at home) or do thoroughly (if you are going out). Brush out your hair carefully.

6.45 p.m.: Dress in a *kaftan* or housegown if you are staying at home or put on your favourite evening clothes if you are going out.

7.30 p.m.: Take a light meal at home. Have fruit juice or half a grapefruit without sugar with two green vegetables. A piece of fresh fruit or fruit salad can also accompany your meal at this time. Tea or coffee with milk but without sugar.

8.30 p.m.: Relax with a magazine or book (Television is not recommended this evening).

10.00 p.m.: Go to bed so that your body and mind get complete rest to wake up fresh and bright, the next morning.

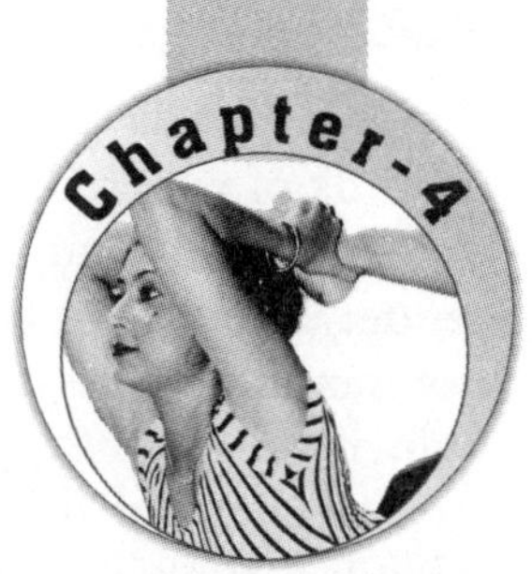

Integumentary System of Human Body

The Integumentary System consists of the skin, hair and nails. It provides the body with a waterproof protective outer covering that contributes to the harmonious working of the whole body. The outermost layer of the skin is called the **epidermis**, beneath which lies the **dermis** and finally, the **hypodermis**. The *hair and nail are extensions of the skin.*

The hypodermis consists of a layer of **fatty tissue**. The **muscles**, **bones** and the various **organs** of the body lie below these layers. The hypodermis is also known as the **subcutaneous layer** or the **subcutis** and is made up of *connective tissue:* **Areolar and Adipose**.

The areolar tissue forms a loose network of cells which provides strength and elasticity to support the blood vessels and the nerve endings.

The adipose tissue forms a network of fat cells to keep our body warm as well as act as a source of energy. Too much body fat caused by over eating as well as too little body fat also put pressure on the body as it loses its energy reserves and heat insulation.

History of the skin

The layer of the skin lying directly *above the hypodermis* is the *dermis* or *true skin.* The cells of the dermis that connect with the hypodermis underneath form the **connective tissue** making up two distinct layers—the *deeper reticular layer* and the *more superficial papillary layer.* The reticular layer contains various types of protein fibres including **collagen, elastin** and **reticulin**. The collagen fibres give the skin strength, resilience and a youthful appearance. Elastin fibres give the skin elasticity enabling it to stretch in order to accommodate an increase in fat cells. Stretch marks occur when elastin fibres fail to respond efficiently to this increase. Reticulin fibres provide support for the many structures held within this layer that include the *hair follicles, sebaceous glands, sweat glands, Arrector pili muscles, nerve supply and circulatory vessels.* Hair follicles are tube-like structures within which hair develop and grow. The hair extend up and out onto the skin through a pore—a minute opening in the skin surface. Each follicle has a rich supply of blood feeding the cells. Sebaceous glands are generally attached to hair follicles and produce the skin's natural lubricant—an oily substance called sebum. The sebum provides lubrication for the skin and the hair, maintaining suppleness and hair lustre. As we comb or brush our hair, the sebum is taken down its length. Remember, brushing the hair one hundred times a day and night would keep it in good condition. The use of heat in the form of hair dryer, evaporates the sebum reducing its lubricating qualities. We replace the lost or lacking sebum with hair conditioners.

Sweat glands are also exocrine glands and are collectively known as **Sudoriferous glands** of which there are two types—*Eccrine* and *Apocrine.* The Eccrine glands are found all over the body but are more numerous on the palms of the hands, the soles of the feet and under the arms. Their function is to produce sweat which helps to regulate the body temperature. The sweat from these glands travels to the surface of the skin via a **sweat duct**, which opens onto a **sweat pore**. Apocrine glands are found mainly in the underarm and genital areas of the body and usually develop in puberty. The sweat produced from these glands is broken down by bacteria present on the surface of the skin, resulting in body odour. Arrector pili muscles are small structures attached to the hair follicles. The tiny muscles contract as the body temperature drops from 36.8° Celsius. The nerve supply in our body involves a complex network of nervous tissue that links the skin with the nervous system. Circulatory vessels are situated throughout this layer linking the skin with the blood and lymph supply of the body. Blood vessels are responsible for feeding the cells with oxygen brought in from the respiratory system. Lymph vessels help to release the waste that collects as a result of this activity.

The epidermis (the uppermost section of the skin) is made up of five main layers of cells which collectively form the **Stratified Epithelial Tissue**. The individual layers of cells are referred to as **Stratum**. The five layers include:

(a) The deepest layer known as *stratum germinativum* or 'basal layer', in which the cells are very active, receiving a rich blood supply from the underlying papillary layer of the dermis. These cells produce new cells, and the old cells are pushed up towards the skin's surface and they enter the next four layers. The process takes about one month to be completed.

- **Keratinocytes:** These produce a protein called 'keratin'.
- **Langerhans cells:** They absorb foreign bodies passing them deeper into the skin.
- **Star shaped cells:** These are also known as **melanocytes** and they produce the colour pigment called *melanin.* Melanin is produced in abundance in dark skins providing the added protection, and is totally lacking in *albino skins.* The ultraviolet rays of the sun activate the increased production within the melanocytes causing the additional melanin to rise, darkening the skin and producing a sun tan.

(b) The old cells are pushed upward forming the next layer, *stratum spinosum* or 'prickle cell layer' consisting of eight layers of cells.

(c) The cells continue to move upwards forming the *stratum granulosum* or the 'granular layer' made up of two to five layers of diamond shaped cells. The destruction of melanin by enzymes begins in this layer of the skin.

(d) The next layer is called *stratum lucidum* or 'clear layer', which consists of several layers of flat, hard cells that contribute the waterproofing function of the skin.

(e) The final layer, i.e., *stratum corneum* or the 'horny layer' consists of up to 25 layers of flat, hard cells that provide the visual appearance of the skin, although the cells of the underlying layers contribute to their overall condition. A good supply of blood to the deeper layer will ensure efficient cell reproduction.

How does skin protect the body

The skin protects the body like a living suit of armour, keeping the vital organs safely in and the environmental enemies out. The protective covering of the skin formed by the combination of the sebum, sweat and the dead skin cells helps to maintain a slightly acidic pH of between 4.6 to 6, depending upon the area of the body. Excessive exposure to the sun will result in premature ageing of the skin. Hair, too, develops from the hair follicles in the dermis and protrudes out on to the surface of the skin. The **terminal hair** offers the skin an additional protection in more delicate areas on the body with a thicker growth and the **vellus hair** growth is in other areas. The skin also contributes to maintain a normal body temperature of 36.8° C with the help of sweating, vasodilation, vasoconstriction, fat cells, etc.

The skin can be divided into seven categories

- **Normal skin** has a fine texture, is supple, smooth, moist, neither greasy nor dry and has smooth pores.
- **Dry skin** has a tendency to flake easily, is prone to lines and wrinkles, retains moisture and ages faster.
- **Oily skin** causes over-secretion of sebum, is prone to pimples, acne, wrinkles, spots and blemishes.
- **Dehydrated skin** lacks moisture, causes wrinkles and premature ageing.
- **Sallow skin** is pale. This is due to deficient diet and lack of vitamin B.
- **Combination skin** has dry and oily patches. Usually cheeks and throat are dry while forehead, nose and chin are oily.
- **Sensitive skin,** also called as hypersensitive or allergic skin, reacts violently. Usually cheeks become red-veined easily or become sore and chapped. For others, the skin may become blotchy, puffy or irritated.

Nerves of the skin

The skin contains many nerve fibres which provide the body with the sense of touch, pain, heat, cold, pressure or deep touch. The pliability of the skin depends upon the elasticity of the dermis. Ageing of the skin is caused as a result of the skin's loss of elasticity. The colour of the skin whether fair, medium or dark depends on the blood supply to the skin and primarily on **melanin**. The melanin protects the sensitive cells of the skin from sunburn and tanning by the ultra-violet rays of the sun. The skin has the following main functions:

- **Protection:** It protects the body from injury or bacterial invasion.
- **Sensation:** It stimulates the sensory nerve endings.
- **Heat regulation:** It protects the body from the environment. A healthy body maintains an internal temperature of 36.8°C..
- **Excretion:** The body excretes perspiration through the skin.

- **Secretion:** The sebaceous glands secrete sebum or oil that lubricate the skin.
- **Absorption:** It occurs when the ingredient enters the body through the skin and the opening of the hair follicles as well as the sebaceous glands.

Basic factors to maintain balance of the skin

The skin, hair and nails will benefit from drinking fluids. Drink as much water as you can at room temperature to aid digestion. Vitamin A, C and E are essential natural anti-oxidants which provide protection to the skin, hair and nails. Take a balanced diet, fresh vegetables and fruits which will contribute to a clear skin, shiny hair and healthy nails. Rest is equally important for the skin cells. An adult needs 6-8 hours of quality sleep in every 24 hours. Rest allows the body and the skin to replenish and regenerate efficiently. Physical activity stimulates the circulation ensuring an active blood supply to the skin. Cleansing, exfoliating, stimulating, toning, applying masks for nourishing, moisturising, etc., are important skin care routines.

Hormones and skin beauty

There is a relationship between beauty and hormones. Lack of or excess of hormones or their imbalance can prove disastrous. Hormones are of various types, but those which affect the skin and beauty are **Androgens, Estrogens, Thyroids, Steroids, Insulin** and **Sex hormones**.

- **Androgens:** These are basically **male hormones**. The excessive secretion causes acne and hair loss due to stress and mental tension.
- **Estrogens**: These are **female hormones** produced by the ovaries. They help to cure acne and pimples, wrinkles and premature ageing, especially after the age of 40. Do not forget to consult a doctor before the treatment of skin lesions, pigmentation of skin and if suffering from high blood pressure.
- **Thyroids:** The shortage of thyroid hormones causes dry skin and wrinkles.
- **Steroids:** The exessive production of thyroid hormones causes skin infections, pigmentation and acne.
- **Insulin:** The deficiency of insulin causes skin fungus, bacterial infection, itching and poor complexion.
- **Sex Hormones:** Male sex hormones enhance the growth of hair on the skin and body, whereas the female sex hormones increase the growth of hair on the scalp.

Hair

Hair develops from the hair follicles and is present on the body prior to the birth, developing as *lanugo hair.* This hair, shortly after birth, is replaced with *vellus hair.* The areas of the body requiring additional protection develop *terminal hair.*

Lanugo hair is soft, fine hair covering the body. *Vellus hair* is soft and downy covering the whole body except for palms of the hand, soles of the feet, the lips and parts of genital areas.

Terminal hair is the coarse hair of the scalp, inside the ears, the eyebrows and eyelashes, underarms and pubic regions.

Hair growth is reliant on hormonal balance and changes occur when this balance is altered. Hormonal changes are responsible for the development of terminal hair from vellus hair, initiating stronger, coarser hair growth in certain areas of the body. Puberty changes hair growth in teenagers. Pregnancy can activate hair growth making it thicker in certain areas of the body, i.e., the abdomen. Menopause can activate male characteristic hair growth in women. Other factors which affect hair growth may include excessive stress levels, heredity and illness.

The growth of lanugo and vellus hair are from the sebaceous glands situated in the dermis, and the terminal hair growth begins at the base of the hair follicles. The hair bulb offers the hair-producing cells a rich supply of blood and nerves. The lower portion of the hair bulb contains the matrix or hair root. The cells within the matrix reproduce new cells by mitosis, pushing old cells upwards in the same way as the cells in the layers of the epidermis. Hair on the head may last up to six years before falling out, yet individual eyelashes fall out after only six months. The follicles produce one hair each, which is made up of **three layers**—the **medulla** (innermost layer made up of loose cells), the **cortex keratinocytes** and **melanocytes** are found in this layer determining the strength and colour of the hair) and the **cuticle** (outermost layer made up of flat overlapping cells).

Individual hair can grow up to half an inch a month. They have a growth cycle which takes them through three stages—**Anagen, the first stage** of hair growth is initiated by the **endocrine system** releasing hormones into the blood stream. The hair cells receive nourishment from the **dermal papilla**. **Catagen** is **the second stage** of growth which involves the hair cells passing up through the follicles. **Tologen** is the **third stage** of growth and the final phase of the cycle. In this stage, the hair dries up and eventually falls out where the fresh hair grows.

Composition of hair

The chemical composition of hair usually varies with the colour of the hair. But generally, it is as follows:

Carbon	:	51%
Hydrogen	:	6%
Nitrogen	:	17%
Oxygen	:	21%
Sulphur	:	5%

The average monthly growth of hair varies between ¼ to ½ inch and the growth is maximum between the ages 20 to 30. The growth is faster in summer than in winter. The life of hair is cyclical, i.e., after a few years of growth, the hair becomes inactive and dies, and then it falls. The life span of a hair can be anything from several months to several years depending upon the health of the scalp. There are **four types of hair**: *Normal, Greasy, Dry* and *Greasy dry.*

Nails

The other external structures of the skin are the nails that develop from cells within the epidermis and protrude to cover the ends of the fingers and toes as hardened plates. Nails do not have a growth cycle like hair. They grow continuously throughout life starting from the third month of foetal development. Nails grow approximately 4 cm per year, growing faster in the summer than in winter. The structure of a nail includes:

- **Germinal matrix**, the root of the nail forms the cell which will eventually produce a nail.
- **Lunula,** a half moon shaped nail plate at the base of the nail that gradually hardens through keratinisation.
- **Nail plate,** which consists of three layers of clear cells and develops with the layers of epidermis forming an extension of the skin at the end of the fingers and the toes. Remember, the nail plate itself is dead and does not bleed or hurt when cut, just like hair.
- **Nail bed** lies directly below the nail plate and is responsible for securing the nail to the finger or toe. The cells of the surface of the **nail bed** interlock with the cells of the underside of the **nail plate**.
- **Free edge** is the part of the nail plate at the end which extends over the nail bed.
- **Nail cuticle**, which develops as an extension of the stratum corneum creating the **nail fold**. It starts as the eponychium at the lanula, attaching itself to the nail plate and protects the underlying germinal matrix against damage and invasion. It surrounds the nail plate as the **peronychium**, extending under the top of the nail plate as the **hyponychium**, and it offers protection to the nail bed.
- **Nail grooves** guide up the fingers and toes at the sides.
- **Nail wall**, the skin which covers the sides of the nail plate protecting the nail grooves.
- **Nail mantle** is the skin lying above the germinal matrix.

Structure of nails

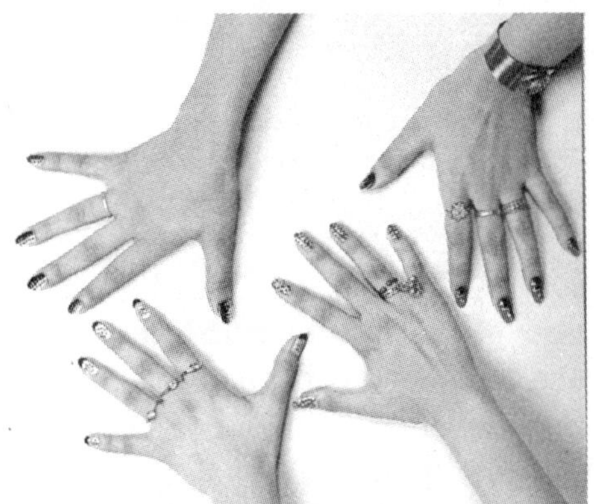

The condition of nails, like that of the skin reflects the general health of the body. The healthy nail is firm, flexible and slightly pink in colour with smooth, curved and unspotted surface. The nail is composed of mainly **keratin** (a protein substance that forms the base of all horny tissue). The horny nail plate contains no nerves or blood vessels. *The nail consists of three parts—the nail body, the nail root and the free edge.*

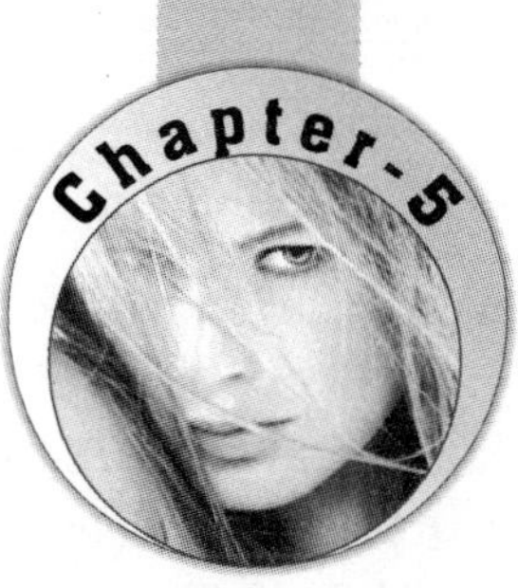

Conditions Affecting the Skin, Hair and Nail

Skin Problems

- **Abscess:** A local infection which is painful, swollen and contains pus formation.
- **Acne Rosacea:** Redness of the nose and cheeks caused by the dilation of the minute capillaries in the skin. Papules and pustules accompany this disorder.
- **Acne Vulgaris:** Infected sebaceous glands resulting in papules, pustules and comedones. Commonly affected areas include the face, neck, back and chest.
- **Allergy:** Sensitivity causing the skin to react adversely which becomes red, hot and itchy.
- **Alopecia:** Baldness in patches on the scalp known as *Alopecia Areata*, or a total hair loss is known as *Alopecia Totalis.* Total hair loss from the whole body is called *Alopecia Universalis.*
- **Asteatosis:** A condition due to under activity of the sebaceous glands causing excessively dry, scaly and itchy skin.
- **Skin Tag:** Tiny, loose growth of skin on the neck or groin. It is colourless and painless. Sometimes, the disorder attacks the armpits and trunks at any age but most commonly in elderly women.
- **Spider Naevus:** Small, painless, red spot with thin blood vessels that usually appear on the face, body and legs during pregnancy.
- **Strawberry Naevus:** A bright red mark varying from a small pinhead to a swollen, irregular dome-shaped mark, most commonly found on the head and the neck.
- **Stretch mark:** Thin lines of over-stretched skin. These are generally shiny and discoloured due to the loss of elasticity in the dermis.
- **Sunburn:** Inflammation of the skin after an excessive exposure to sun.
- **Superfluous hair:** Unwanted hair as a result of heredity, hormonal changes or due to stimulation in a particular area.
- **Urticaria (Hives):** Characterised by a swollen area of the skin surrounded by a red wheal.
- **Vitiligo:** White patches of the skin caused by destruction of melanocytes. It is caused mostly due to hormonal imbalance.
- **Warts:** Small, solid growth on the skin caused by a virus. Highly contagious. When they appear on the feet, they are known as *Veruccas.*

- **Wheal:** A localised area of swelling.
- **Whitlow:** An infection at the tip of the finger or thumb. It is generally tender to touch with a pus formation.

Dry skin

If your skin feels tight, looks dull and flaky—it is a dry skin. A dry skin is prone to wrinkles and premature ageing. If your skin problem has become widespread and uncomfortable and there is no improvement after two weeks of self-care, see a dermatologist for diagnosis and treatment. The following steps should be adopted to treat a dry skin:

- Aromatherapy treatment: A warm facial compress, using essential oils greatly benefits a dry skin. Fill a basin with lukewarm water and add to it two to three drops of one of the three essential oils: lavender, rose or neroli.
- Do not apply soap to wash the facial skin. Use a washing gel.
- Follow each bath with a moisturiser.
- Drink 7–8 glasses of water a day to keep the skin hydrated and prevent dryness.
- Use oatmeal as a soap substitute. Oatmeal is a soothing agent.
- Beta-carotene taken with lunch and dinner is a nutrient diet for soft, smooth, disease-free skin. (Normal dose—15 milligrams a day taken half, twice each with lunch and dinner).
- Mineral Zinc (15 milligrams daily dose) is an important nutrient for the repair of damaged skin tissue. Zinc deficiency can cause dry skin.
- Vitamin B complex (100 milligrams a day) cures a dry skin and other skin diseases.
- Vitamin C (1,000 milligrams a day) helps the immune system, which leads to a healthier skin.
- Vitamin E capsules (400 international units a day) is a strong nutrient for the skin, which helps replace cells on the skin's outer layer.

Oily skin

An oily skin having medium to large pores on the skin has the following symptoms:

- Blackheads and acnes.
- Is prone to skin blemishes.

Treatment to get rid of oily skin:

- Aromatherapy treatments can be very beneficial for oily skin to help balance glandular activity, improve circulation and detoxify.
- Steaming helps to deep-cleanse oily skin. Steam the face once a week. Start cleaning the face with soap followed by steaming. Next, rinse with warm water and finally, splash with cool water and pat dry.

- Keep your muscles loose.
- Gentle Yoga exercise and Chinese exercises of Tai Chi help build your energy.
- Avoid watching TV as far as possible, which makes one lethargic. Try reading instead, that energises.
- Think positive, be motivated and be confident. These thoughts affect your energy level.
- Breathe deeply. It makes you relaxed and energised.
- Avoid sleeping pills.
- The colour on the walls of your house leaves a good effect on your mind. Dark colours make you feel fatigued. Red colour is good for short-term energy stimulation. Green colour is good at eliminating fatigue.
- Light music helps fight fatigue.

Dry hair

Like skin, dry hair looks lifeless, lacking lustre and may be brittle with split ends. The hair becomes dry as a result of too much sun exposure, blow drying or chemical treatments such as colouring and perms. When hair becomes dry, the outer layer called cuticle peels off from the central shaft. Use hair conditioner to lubricate the hair and prevent static electricity. Beer is a wonderful hair setting lotion to give a crisp, healthy, shiny look to dry hair.

Oily hair

Oily hair is caused by overly oily scalp and one common cause of an oily scalp is a high-fat diet. The hair is fed through hair bulbs in the scalp, which are intertwined with sebaceous glands that produce oil, also known as sebum. A diet full of fried foods and saturated fats can trigger over-production of sebum. Those women with fine hair have as many as 1,40,000 oil glands on their scalp. Redheads have an average 80,000 to 100,000 hair on the scalp. To decrease the oil production from the scalp and reduce oiliness, the following remedies are suggested:

- Rinse hair with lemon water after shampooing. Squeeze juice of two lemons into two cups of soft water. Apply this liquid evenly to your hair and massage gently. Leave it for five minutes, then rinse with cool to tepid water. Blot your hair dry with a towel.
- Use of the herb horsetail is an effective remedy for oily hair. Boil one cup of distilled water, adding to it 2 tablespoons of dried powder of horsetail. Use liquid as a last rinse after shampoo.
- Aromatherapy also helps to reduce the oil in hair. Add 3-4 drops of rosemary, lavender, eucalyptus, cypress or lemon oil in rinsing water. All these oils are astringent and cleanse and tone the sebaceous glands.
- Massage your scalp gently during the shampoo.

- Don't over-brush your hair as brushing from the roots carries oil from the scalp to the ends of the hair.
- Learn to relax. When you are under stress, the body produces more androgens, which produce excessive oil.
- Apply astringent to the scalp, which helps to slow down the oil secretion from the scalp.

Hair loss

Hair loss in women is difficult to diagnose and can be caused by many factors as below:

- Alopecia areata (baldness on the scalp in patches).
- Hormone imbalances.
- Effect of menopause.
- Shortage of dietary protein and amino acid deficiency.
- Intestinal parasites.
- Damage from hair treatments.
- Stress and sudden shock.
- After-effect of a fever.
- Effect of childbirth.

Consult a doctor for suitable treatment, if hair continues falling even after a treatment. The following measures are suggested:

- **Aromatherapy:** Essential oils such as jojoba oil, rosemary oil, lavender oil, lemon balm and cedar wood oil helps fight hair loss. Massage the mixture into the scalp with your fingertips. Leave it on for 30 minutes or overnight, then shampoo in the morning. As a final rinse, add one drop of lavender oil and one drop of rosemary oil to ½ litre water and pour it over the head.
- You may consult an experienced beauty therapist for suitable advice to maintain your hair.

Diseases of hair

Dandruff: It is sometimes loosely scattered in the hair. The other waxy or greasy type of dandruff is yellow scaliness mixed with sebum which sticks to the scalp causing itchiness. If the greasy scales are torn off, bleeding or oozing of sebum may follow. On the slightest sign of dandruff, treat it without delay.

To fight dandruff, mix two tablespoons of cosmetic vinegar and six tablespoons of water. Dab with cotton into the scalp, parting the hair with a comb. Preferably apply it at bed time. Tie a scarf over the head to avoid staining the bed clothes. Wash the hair with shampoo the next morning. Rinse your hair thoroughly and pour over a last rinse–a mixture of three tablespoons of cosmetic vinegar and a cup of hot water. Hot oil therapy is another method to cure dandruff. Massage hot oil into the scalp at bedtime. Next morning, rub lemon juice mixed with cosmetic vinegar into the scalp with cotton wool. Give the hair a good wash with egg shampoo followed by a last rinse of a mixture of the juice of one lemon in a cup of hot water. Continue this treatment once or twice a week for three months. Giving the hair and the scalp a hot steam bath is a magical cure to treat dandruff. Massage hot oil and wrap a hot damp towel on the head like a turban to enable the steam fight dandruff.

Alopecia — The round patches on the scalp

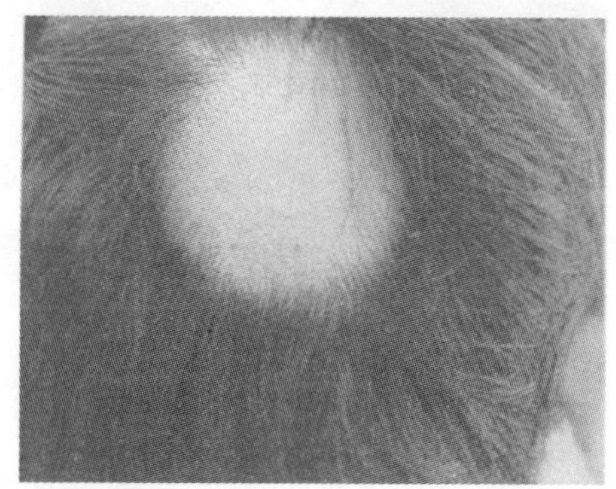

The sudden appearance of small bald patches on the scalp is a matter of worry. The situation can be alarming if these patches grow larger and join up. Alopecia is generally of three types:

- **Alopecia Senilis** which usually occurs in old age. The hair loss is permanent.
- **Alopecia Premature** occurs any time before middle age by a slow thinning process.
- **Alopecia Aerata** is sudden baldness in round patches, occurring at young age.

Treatments include massaging the scalp with remains of tobacco from the 'hookah' in mustard oil, stimulating the blood circulation of the scalp by friction with tincture of cantharides or potassium permanganate lotion and applying carbonic snow (dry ice) on bald patches, which gives an alternate cold and hot feeling.

Ringworm and Eczema

One or several round-shaped grey coloured patches appearing on the scalp, usually among children, are ringworms. This contagious scalp disease is caused by a certain type of fungi. There are two main groups of ringworms: the **Shearing Ringworm** and the **Favus Ringworm**. The first type is most common in India and forms bald patches but this is not a permanent loss of hair. The **Favus Ringworm** is rare, only found in slum areas having poor hygienic conditions. This type of ringworm is most dangerous and it attacks the bulb as well as the hair causing permanent baldness. If untreated, the patches become larger and join each other. Consult a doctor immediately for treatment. Cut the hair short to make treatment easier and cover the hair with a cap.

Do you feel itchy on the scalp? If so, you are suffering from **eczema**. An itchy scalp can be caused by inadequate rinsing after shampooing, effect of chlorine, salt and chemicals in hair cosmetic preparations. To cure eczema, use a vinegar rinse after shampooing. Wash your hair every other day with a very mild shampoo followed by lemon or vinegar rinse. Use a scalp conditioner regularly. Bergamot *(zabir)*, nettle *(bichchhubooti)*, parsley *(ajmod)*, thyme *(ban ajwain)*, rosemary *(rusemari)*, yarrow *(gahastrapani or gandana)* and raspberry leaves heal and soothe this condition. Sunflower oil and olive oil heated with rosemary or nettle alleviates an itchy scalp. Egg shampoo mixed with orange juice is a magic remedy for oily hair and an itchy scalp. Apply it to the hair and leave for ten minutes, then rinse thoroughly with lukewarm water.

Premature Grey Hair

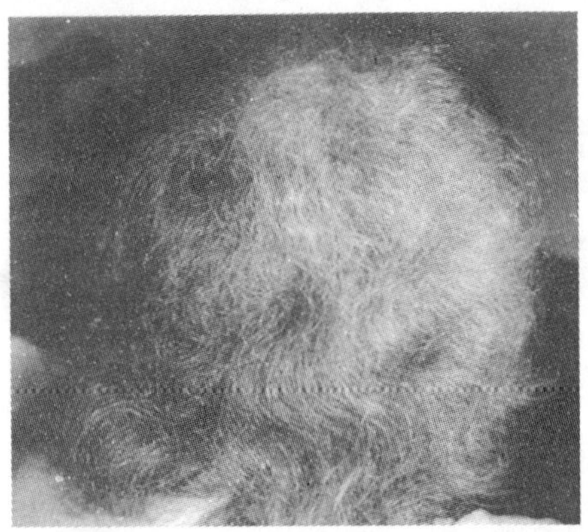

The things have changed now, in the past, grey hair were symbolic of old age to signify seniority and experience. Today, most of the young men and women are suffering from premature greying of hair and hence, are left with no option but to dye their hair. Premature greying of hair signifies some deficiency in the body as well as polluted atmosphere, unhygienic circumstances, scorching heat and sultry climate. Tension, anxiety, grief, disease, worry and frustration—are harmful for the beauty of hair and promote premature greying. *Henna* is a popular herbal dye to give a reddish brown tinge.

Hair dandruff (seborrhoeic dermatitis)

Scalp irritation?

Thick scale, despite regular use of dandruff shampoo?

Yellow crusting?

Red patches along the neckline?

Itchiness?

If the reply is 'yes', you are suffering from hair dandruff. There are many possible causes of dandruff, including a yeast infection of the scalp or hormone imbalances. If all the treatments to cure dandruff fail, consult a dermatologist for proper diagnosis and medical treatment. If you have dandruff, do not use dandruff shampoos. Instead, treat your scalp with the essential oils of aromatherapy. Dandruff is not a hair problem, but a skin problem. The flaking and itchiness are the result of an over-production of a substance called sebum from the glands in the scalp. These glands are usually hyperactive because of excessively dry hair. Hair shampoos available in the market for the treatment of dandruff and strong medications to control it, however, may provide a temporary relief but they don't do anything to address the underlying disorder such as dryness and poor health of the scalp. Such dandruff shampoos and strong medicines destroy the scalp's delicate balance of water and oil, which irritated the glands. The following natural ways stop flaking:

- **Aromatherapy** helps to eliminate dandruff.

  Collect the following ingredients:

Unscented mild shampoo	2 tablespoons
Tea tree oil	10 drops
Cedar wood oil	8 drops
Pine oil	6 drops
Rosemary oil	6 drops
Clary sage oil	4 drops
Lemon oil	4 drops

  Mix the above ingredients. These essential oils encourage the body's system to heal the problems that cause dandruff. Tea tree oil is an antiseptic helping to normalise the bacteria on the scalp. Rosemary and cedar wood oil increase circulation in the scalp. Pine oil encourages elimination of toxins from the skin of the scalp. Clary sage helps regulate and balance the oil production and lemon encourages elimination of toxins and promotes internal cleansing. Use shampoo several times a week.

- **Massage:** Dandruff is a symptom of a body-wide condition of 'vata' or dryness, Massaging the scalp twice a week with warm sesame oil combats the excessive dryness. It is also very calming and soothing to the system, which is important, since dandruff is often caused by anxiety. Massage the oil into your scalp before sleep for about ten minutes. Then wrap your head with a hot towel and steam the face for ten minutes. Wash the hair next morning.
- **Vitamin E:** This helps to balance the oils on the scalp and relieves dryness, (recommended dose a capsule of 400 IU a day).
- **Zinc:** It helps your scalp heal from dandruff. This mineral rebuilds the skin (recommended dose 15-20 milligrams daily).
- **Selenium** relieves flaking and itching due to dandruff, (recommended dose 200-microgram supplement daily).
- **Eucalyptus** rinse helps fight infection due to dandruff. To make a rinse, put 4 teaspoons of dried leaves in half a litre boiling water and stir. Then cover, remove from heat and keep for an hour. Strain the liquid and add to it 1 tablespoon of apple-cider vinegar. After taking a shower, pour the rinse very slowly over the hair, but do not rinse it out, just let it dry.

Nail irregularities

- **Corrugation:** These are wavy ridges caused by the uneven growth of nails due to illness or an injury. Buff the nails with pumice power. This helps to remove or minimise the ridges.

- **Furrows:** Depression in the nails run lengthwise or across the nails due to illness or an injury to the nail. Avoid the use of metal pusher. A cotton tipped orangewood stick should be used around the cuticle.
- **White spots:** These spots do not indicate a disease caused by an injury. As the nail continues to grow, these white spots eventually disappear. These are also called as Leuconychia.
- **Hypertrophy:** An overgrowth of the nails in thickness rather than lengthwise caused by local infection or hereditary factor. In case of an infection, do not manicure the nails.
- **Atrophy of the nail:** Atrophy or wasting away of the nail causes the nail to lose its lustre and sometimes become shorter or is shed entirely. It is also called as Onychotrophia.
- **Pterygium:** Growth of the cuticle sticking to the base of the nail and is generally caused by circulatory problem.
- **Onychophagy:** Bitten nails caused due to an acquired nervous habit that hardens the cuticle.
- **Onychorrhexis:** Split or brittle nails due to careless filing, deficiency of vitamins, illness, effect of strong soap and water, excessive use of cuticle solvents and nail polish remover. A manicure is recommended.
- **Hangnail:** A common condition in which the cuticle splits around the nail and causes the dryness or due to cutting off the cuticle carelessly. If not taken care, a hangnail may become infected. It is also called as Agnail.
- **Eggshell nails:** Such nails have thin, white nail plate and are more flexible than a normal nail. The nail plate separates from the nail bed and curves at the free edges. This is caused by chronic illness.
- **Blue nails:** It is caused by poor blood circulation or a heart disease. A regular manicure is recommended.
- **Bruised nail:** These are dark, purplish (almost black or brown) spots usually due to an injury or bleeding in the nail bed. The dried blood attaches itself to the nail and grows.
- **Treating cut:** This is usually caused during a careless manicure. To protect against infection, apply a sterile bandage or an antiseptic.
- **Infected finger:** The patient should be referred to a doctor.
- **Fungus mould:** Fungi is the general term for a vegetable parasite. Fungi and nail mould both are contagious. They can spread from one nail to the other nail.
- **Nail fungus:** A discolouration in the nail which spreads towards the cuticle. Fungus may affect the hands, feet and must be referred to a doctor.

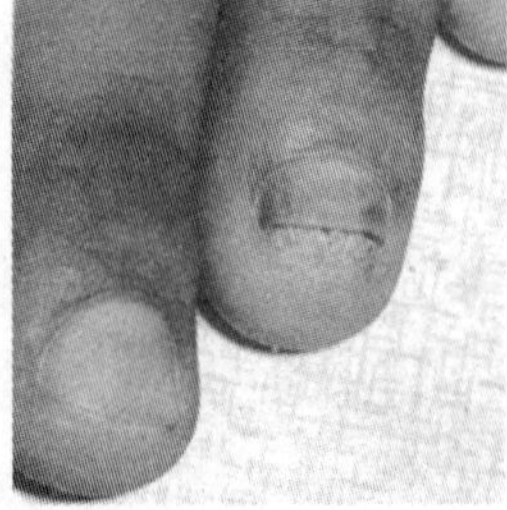

- **Nail mould:** A fungus infection caused when the moisture is trapped between the unsaphitised natural nail and products that are put over the nail. A nail mould can be identified in the early stages as yellow or green spots that become darker in advance stages if the nail has been infected. The discolouration becomes black gradually and the nail softens and smells bad. The nail problem should be consulted with a doctor immediately before it falls off.

Diseases of nails and feet

There are several nail diseases that one may suffer from. Any nail disease that shows signs of infection or inflammation such as redness, pain and swelling must not be treated in a beauty saloon. It should be referred to a doctor. Infection occurs in people who regularly expose their hands to soaps, solvents and other chemical materials. Some of the common nail diseases are described below:

- **Onychosis:** A technical term applied to a nail disease is called Onychosis.
- **Onychomycosis:** Also known as *ringworm of the nail.* It is an infection of the nail caused by a fungus. The disease invades the free edge and spreads towards the root. The infected layers peel off and expose the diseased parts at the nail bed.
- **Ringworm of the hands:** It is a highly contagious disease caused by a fungus. The main symptoms are *red lesions* occurring in patches or rings over the hands, with itching.

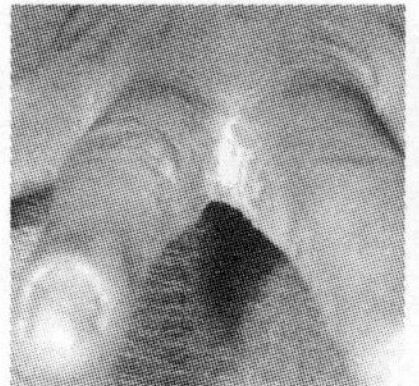

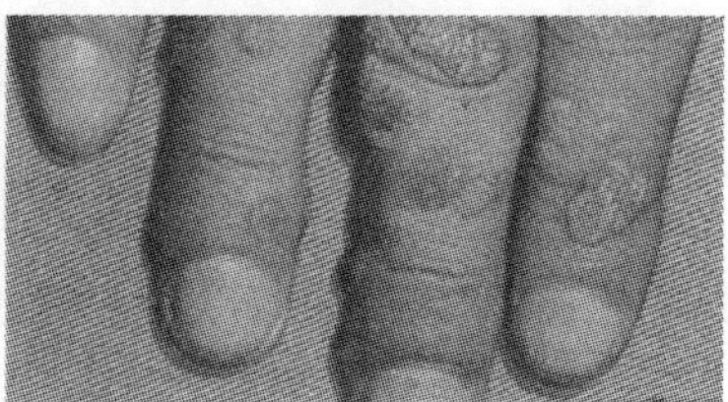

- **Paronychia:** This is also known as Felon, which is an infectious and inflammatory condition of the tissue surrounding the nail. It is also characterised by gradual thickening and brownish discolouration of the nail plate.
- **Onychia:** It is an inflammation of the nail matrix accompanied by pus formation.
- **Ingrown nails:** The nail grows into the sides of the flesh and can cause infection. Ill fitting shoes can also cause ingrown nails.
- **Onychoptosis:** A periodic shedding of one or more nails.
- **Onycholysis:** It is the loosening of the nails without shedding.

Corns and callouses

Corns, common among housewives and working women, are the ugly little bumps and lumps of dead skin cells on the feet as a result of friction and irritation between the feet and shoes. Callouses are your body's way of protecting you from pressure. When the pressure increases, the callous gets thicker and thicker. People having callouses live easily than with painful corns between and on toes.

What to do in case of blisters: The footwear that pinches gives you blisters. Shoes should not be loose, as constant rubbing can also give rise to blisters. The following precautions are essential in case of suffering from blisters:

- Till the blister has dried, do not wear the same shoes.
- Use a talcum powder and keep it dry.
- Cover the blister when you are going out, but otherwise air it properly.
- Use an antiseptic cream over the blister.
- Do not tamper with the blister yourself but consult a doctor.
- Do not try to puncture the blister yourself, it can infect your skin.

If the same defective shoe is being worn repeatedly and a blister is left untreated, you will develop corns. Make sure you change your footwear frequently. Scrub corns hard with a pumice stone and massage thereafter. Usually, the corns on the sole of the feet are painful and give trouble. Better consult a doctor. Never be tempted to remove the corn by attempting to cut it with a pair of scissors.

Cracked nails, sweaty toes, foot odour, enlarged veins, cracked heels, rough skin, tanned toes, swollen feet, bunions and fungal infection are some of common problems in women. Cracked nails often happen as a result of neglecting your toenails. Sweaty toes can pose a lot of problems and acquire a peculiar odour. The following care should be taken:

- Wash your feet with cold water often.
- Use a skin astringent on the soles of your feet.
- Sprinkle a little talcum powder before wearing a closed shoe.
- Do not wear the same shoe everyday.
- Use a strong eau-de-cologne on the toes, as it acts as an anti-perspirant and kills odour too.
- Wear cotton or woollen socks and avoid wearing nylon socks altogether.

Enlarged veins usually appear where one has to stand a lot, and sometimes from wearing high heels. Your feet need a rest. Avoid wearing high heels and ensure that the garters on your nylon stockings are not tight. Cracked heels is a very common complaint in women due to lack of moisture and oil. Prevent cracked heels by using glycerine and oil to massage your feet once a week. If the skin is rough, apply a lanolin based cream and a good moisturiser all over to keep the skin moist.

When one walks around a lot in the sun, the feet acquire a lot of tan. Bleaching can help you get rid of it. Do not expose your feet too much to the sun. Swollen feet happen if one is not used to standing or sitting for too long. Avoid feet hanging down and wearing tight shoes. Wash your feet with hot soapy water. Keep your legs up in the air along the walls for at least five minutes daily. This cures swelling on the feet. Bunions are changes that take place in the bones because of pressure of the shoes on the toes. It is best to prevent such condition from developing.

Feet are more prone to fungus infection, because the fungus infection thrives in a moist and airless atmosphere where the sun doesn't reach. Switch over to open shoes or sandals without socks. Use an anti-fungus cream, especially between the toes—a breeding place for the infection.

Athlete's foot

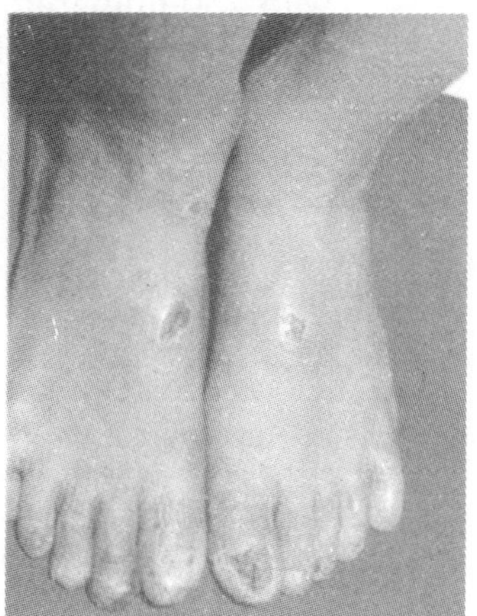

A condition caused by an organism that lives on the skin and breeds under warm and moist conditions. Sweaty footwear is most often responsible for this disorder. This is an acute form of dermatitis. The common symptoms include the following:

- Cracked skin.
- Red, swollen, sore and oozing blisters.
- Intermittent burning sensation.

The inflammation is not dangerous, but it can lead to bacterial infection if not treated properly. The following treatment is recommended:

- Use soothing compresses to cool the inflammation, ease the pain, lessen the itching and dry the sores. Mix two tablespoons of Burrow's solution in ½ litre cold water and apply the solution with cotton cloth, 3–4 times a day.
- Soak your foot in a solution of 2 teaspoons salt mixed to ½ litre water for 5–10 minutes until the problem clears up.
- Apply an anti-fungal cream on your feet as recommended by your doctor.
- To avoid fungus on your feet, especially between the toes, apply a little baking soda paste. To make a paste, mix 1 tablespoon of baking soda to lukewarm water and rub on the site of fungus, then rinse and dry.
- Toenails are the breeding spots for the fungus. Scrape the undersides clean every second or third day with an orangewood stick.
- After the infection has cleared up, apply an anti-fungal cream or lotion regularly.
- Avoid the use of plastic shoes and footwear; they trap perspiration and create a warm, moist spot for the fungus to grow. Keep your feet dry and clean. Give your shoes a little time in the sun to air out.
- Powder your toes frequently.

Consult a doctor immediately in case:

- Inflammation proves incapacitating.
- Swelling occurs in the foot or the leg at any time during the attack, and you develop a fever.
- Pus appears in the blisters or the cracked skin.

- Dab regular, plain yoghurt on the infected areas. The yoghurt helps reduce the symptoms of athlete's foot and is soothing to the skin.
- Rub 2–3 drops of garlic oil on the affected areas of your feet to kill the foot fungus.
- Vitamin C is the best nutrient for strengthening the immune system. Start treatment with 250-milligram capsules for the first week, increase to 500-milligram dosages the second week, and then to 1,000 milligrams in the third week. If you develop diarrhoea or loose bowel movements due to the possible side-effect of large doses of vitamin C, go back to the quantity of dose at which you will not have any loose motions.

The Skin—Different Age Groups

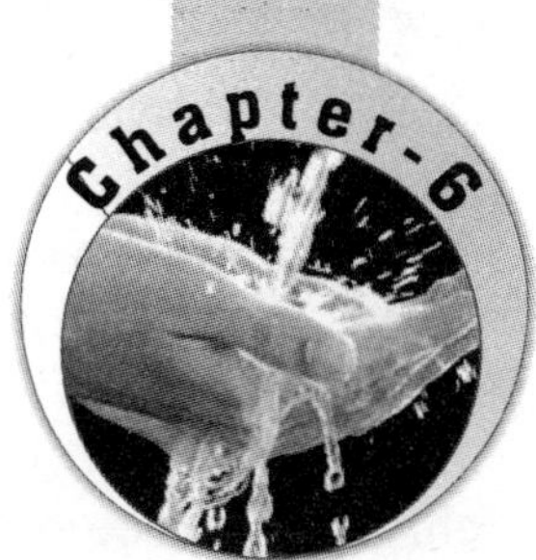

Skin changes with age

Age	Appearance	Physiology
Less than 15	Perfect skin; smooth sebaceous texture.	Excellent repair capabilities; low gland activity; excellent skin hydration.
15-25	Acne and fine lines appear; pore size starts to increase.	High sebaceous gland activity; mild drop in dermal repair; rapid cell turnover; slight drop in skin hydration.
25-45	More fine lines and first wrinkles appear; signs of sagging near the eyes and some loss of elasticity.	Less collagen and increasing accumulation of damaged corrective tissue; drop in skin hydration.
45-55	More wrinkles, rough texture, sallow yellow complexion begins to appear; sagging near the eyes and cheeks.	Continued dermal degradation; cohesion between skin layers continues to decline; thinning of epidermis and the skin tends to be dry.
55 & above	Wrinkles and fine lines in abundance; uneven colour; pigmentation; sagging worsens and dark circles under the eyes.	Compromised dermal repair; abundance of damaged connective tissue; low production of collagen and sebum; increased production of melanin.

Caring for the skin — different age groups

All natural phenomena can have an adverse effect on the skin. Hence, skin care should be adopted according to the change in climate. All skins need care. If neglected, it is prone to several disorders, such as blackheads, whiteheads, steatoma, asteatosis, seborrhoea, pimples, acne vulgaris, bromidrosis, osmidrosis, anidrosis, hyderidrosis, prickly heat, sunburn, inflammations, dermatitis, eczema, ringworm, red veins, lesions, leucoderma, leprosy, burns and scalds, freckles, birthmarks and scars, wrinkles, hirsutism, warts, moles, scabies, boils, blotchiness, odour and fungus infection, psoriasis, melasma, candida, sycosis, barbac, chronic paronychia, intertrigo, herpes, skin tumours, photodermatitis, lichen planus, erytheme multiforme, abscess, acne rosacea, blisters, bed sores (deculatus ulcer), barber's rash (fooliculitis), skin allergy, bruises, skin cancer, cellulitis (spreading inflammation of skin), cherry spots (appear on the chest and trunk), chillblains, cholasma (small dark patches), cold sores (herpes simplex), corns, cysts, crow's feet, fissures, hives (urticaria), genital scabies, impetigo, keloid, kibes, pigmented naevi, port wine stains and macules are some of the chronic skin disorders and allergies which mar many a lovely face. There are a number of herbal preparations for cleansing, moisturising, nourishing, toning and steaming of the skin leaving no after-effect. A badly neglected twenty-year old skin may look more like the complexion of a woman in her late thirties and a woman of thirty plus who has looked after her skin since her teens can well have a skin which fits below the twenty age group.

Age spots

Brown spots start to pepper the backs of your hands when a woman reaches her forties or fifties. They also leave an adverse effect on the facial skin. These are also called as sun spots, as they are generally caused by a direct exposure to the sun's ultra-violet radiation, which damages the colour producing cells of the skin. In fact, age spots are a cosmetic problem, not a medical or health-threatening condition. They can be medically removed by the following methods:

- The process of bleaching.
- Applying liquid nitrogen.
- By laser surgery.
- Consult a doctor if the area around a spot has turned black and irregular in shape. These are signs of melanoma.
- Aromatherapy helps the spot to fade or lighten. The essential oils of lemon have bleaching properties that eliminate the age spot. Add three drops of oil, preferably almond oil and apply the mixture to the spot twice a day for a couple of months.
- A mixture of honey and yoghurt creates a natural bleach that can help to lighten the age spots. To a teaspoon of plain yoghurt, mix thoroughly a teaspoon of honey. Apply this mixture to the hands, let it dry and wash it off after half an hour. Hands are the organs in a human body from where ageing starts.

Skin blemishes

Any kind of spot or number of spots on the face spoil the personality and charm of a woman. Every beauty conscious woman wants to avoid such beauty dampeners. The spots and skin disorders are of various kinds. In case of any skin infection or if suffering from a contagious skin disorder, the matter should be referred to a dermatologist. A **lesion** is a structural change in the tissues caused by an injury or a disease. These are of two types: **primary** and **secondary.**

Primary lesions

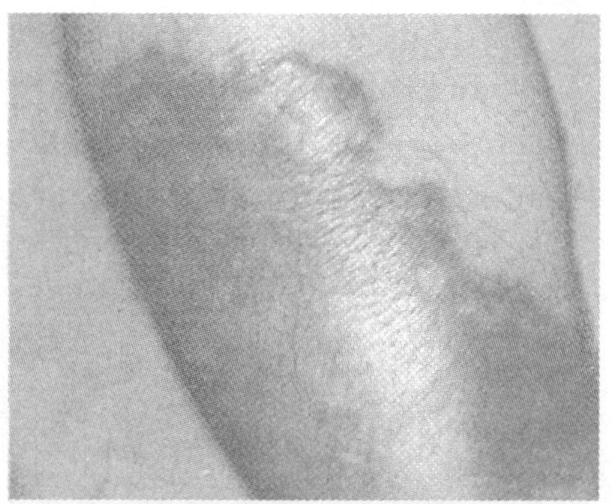

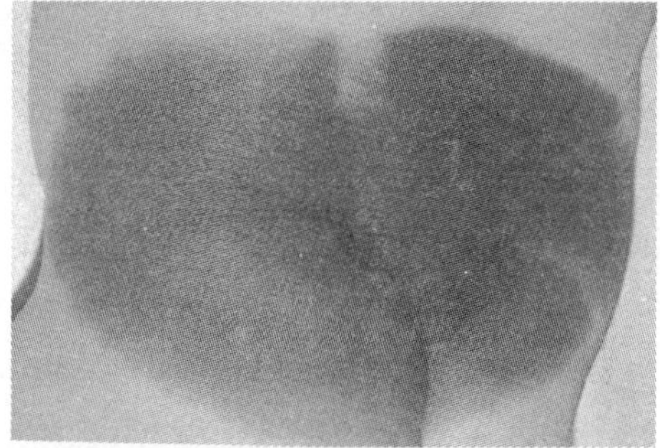

Primary lesions are usually of eight types, such as:

- **Macule** (a small spot on the skin, neither raised nor sunken),
- **Papule** (an elevated pimple developing pus),
- **Wheal** (an itchy, swollen spot usually caused by a mosquito or an insect bite,
- **Tubercle** (a solid lump above or under the surface of the skin, varying in size),
- **Tumour** (an external swelling varying in size, shape and colour),
- **Vesicle** (a small blister containing fluid, beneath the epidermis),
- **Bulla** (a blister containing a watery fluid, smaller to a vesicle) and
- **Pustule** (an elevation of the skin, which contains pus).

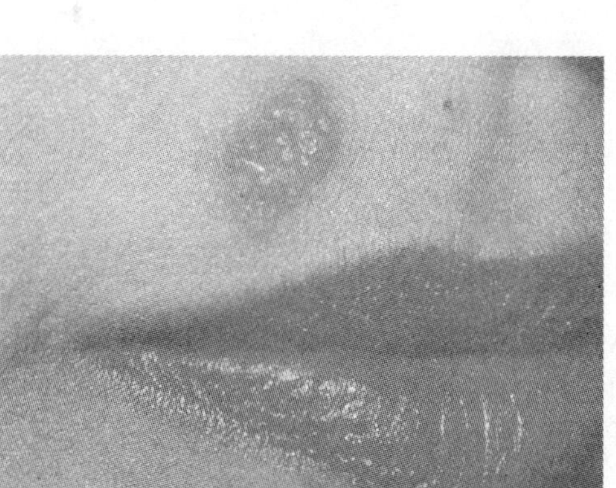

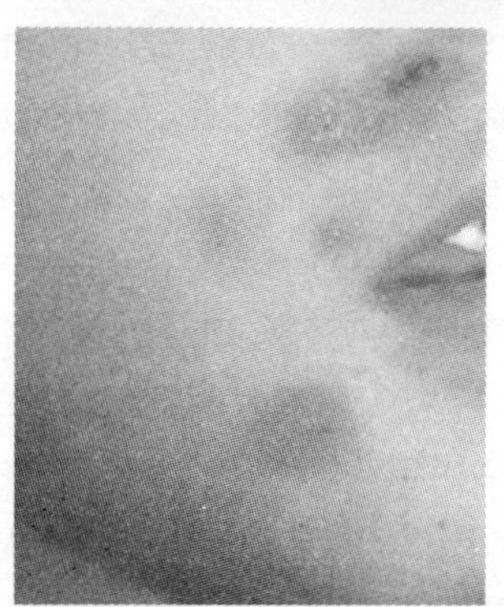

The secondary lesions

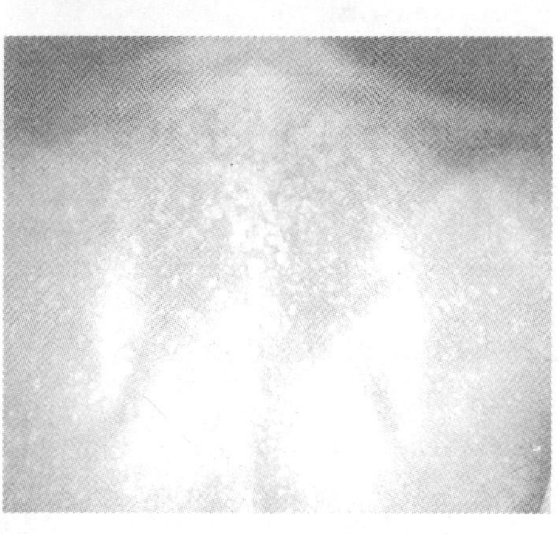

These lesions are serious in nature and are usually of seven types, such as:

- **Scale** (dry or greasy),
- **Crust** or **Scab** (an accumulation of sebum and pus),
- **Excoriation** (a skin abrasion produced by scratching or scraping),
- **Fissure** (a crack in the skin),

- **Ulcer** (an open lesion accompanied by pus),
- **Scar** (formed after an injury) and
- **Stain** (discolouration of the skin).

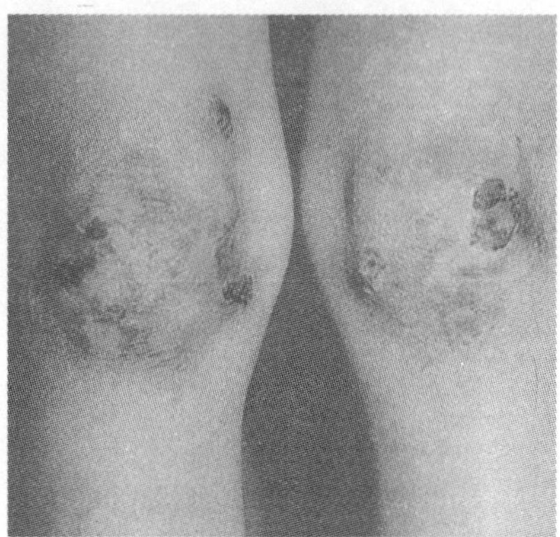

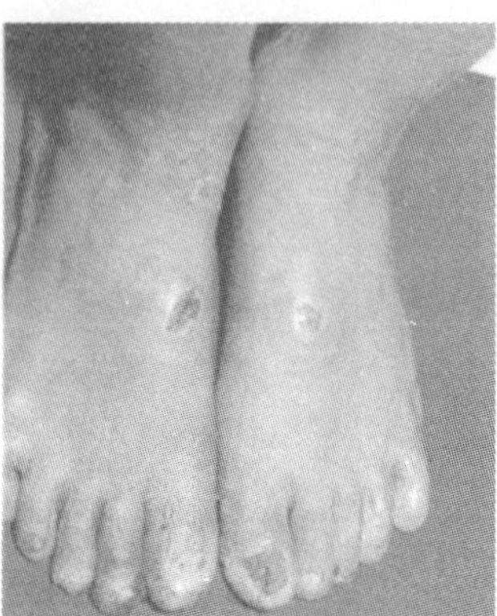

Skin disease is an infection of the skin which is visible and may consist of *scales, pimples* or *pustules.* Some of the common terms applied to skin diseases are:

- **Acute diseases** (less violent and of short duration),
- **Chronic disease** (of long duration),
- **Infectious disease** (caused by pathogenic germs),
- **Contagious disease** (caused by contact),
- **Congenital disease** (present since birth),
- **Seasonal disease** (influenced by the weather),
- **Occupational disease** (afflicted by one's occupation),
- **Parasitic disease** (caused by a vegetable or animal parasite),
- **Pathogenic disease** (produced by bacteria),
- **Systemic disease** (caused by a faulty diet),
- **Venereal disease** (a contagious sex disease acquired by contact with an infected person),
- **Epidemic disease** (disease that attacks a large number of persons in a locality) and
- **Allergy** (a sensitivity developed or caused by contact).

Diseases of glands

These are of two types: **Sebaceous gland diseases** and **Sweat gland diseases**.

Sebaceous gland diseases

These include:

- **Blackheads** (worm-like mass of hardened sebum appearing frequently on the face, forehead and the nose),

- **Whiteheads or Milia** (caused by the accumulation of sebaceous matter beneath the skin on the face, neck, chest and shoulders),
- **Steatoma or Sebaceous cyst** (a subcutaneous tumour filled with sebum varying in size of a pea to that of an orange, on the scalp, neck and back),
- **Asteatosis** (dry, scaly skin, characterised by the deficiency of sebum, generally developing in youth or in old age),
- **Seborrhoea** (due to overactivity and excessive secretion of the sebaceous or oil glands, accompanied by itching or burning sensation generally on the nose, forehead and the scalp) and
- **Acne** (a chronic inflammatory disease occurring frequently on the face, back and the chest).

Sweat gland diseases

Bromidrosis or Osmidrosis (due to foul smell, perspiration, usually noticeable in the armpits or on the feet), **Anidrosis** (due to lack of perspiration), **Hyderidrosis** (due to excessive perspiration, heat or body weakness) and **Miliaria rubra or Prickly heat** (due to exposure to excessive heat).

Bad breath (halitosis)

Remember, brushing and flossing your teeth regularly can clean up some of the oral bacteria that commonly cause bad breath. Chronic type of bad breath may be caused due to many different types of diseases, such as:

- Cancer
- Kidney failure
- Diabetes
- Tuberculosis
- Syphilis (a venereal disease)
- Dehydration
- Zinc deficiency
- Some drugs, including penicillamine and lithium.

To test your breath, cup your hands on the mouth and breathe into them with a great, deep, 'haaaaaa'. Sniff, if it smells bad, then you smell bad. To relieve bad breath, the following measures are taken:

- Rinse your mouth out when you can't brush. After having meals, get a mouthful of water, which will wash the smell of the food from your mouth.
- Eat three meals a day. Often bad breath can be caused by irregular food habits. Bad breath is caused by the side-effects of fasting or by having a poor diet.

- Swallowing water when having meal outside is another method to save from bad breath. You can excuse yourself from the dining table. Take a sip of water and circulate it across and around your teeth. Then swallow bits of food.
- Use tongue scraper. A lot of odour-producing bacteria as well as some smelly, decaying food particles cover the surface of your tongue. Scrape them off with a tongue scraper—a U shaped device, which is dragged over the length of your tongue to collect bacteria and food particles accumulated over the tongue.
- Odorise your digestive tract with chlorophyll, which relieves from bad breath caused by digestive problems in the stomach and intestinal tract and can cause mouth odour.
- Activated charcoal is a natural breath sweetener, which can clean out your insides and sweeten your breath. Take one capsule a day until the problem is solved. If the results are not encouraging, consult a dentist.
- Digestive enzymes break down bad breath. Lack of digestive enzymes causes poor digestion resulting in bad breath.
- Herbs such as ginger, coriander, cumin, aniseed, cloves and fennel are common herbs that can deodorise intestinal tract.

Some Skin Afflictions and Diseases

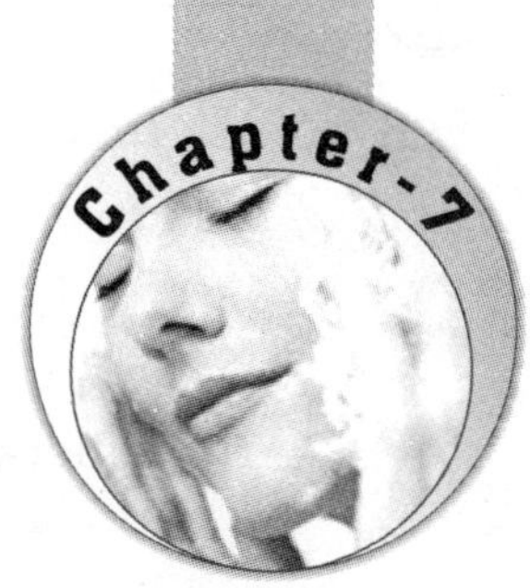

Allergy

Allergy is a state of abnormal sensitivity to a substance or substances. An allergy is what happens when your body detects a foreign substance it doesn't like. Allergies come in almost infinite variety: contact, food or inhalant allergies. The most common causes of allergy are pollen, mould spores, dust, strong fumes, animal hairs, various foods, drugs, serums, anti-toxins, dyes, perfumes, plastics and other chemicals, bites or stings of insects. Symptoms include running nose, nasal stuffiness, wheezing and shortness of breath, red and itchy eyes, sneezing, itching of the skin, swellings, severe rashes, hives, sinus headache, scratchy throat, vomiting, diarrhoea, abdominal cramps and others. Some of the most common allergic diseases are hay fever, bronchial asthma, eczema, hives (urticaria), contact dermatitis and migraine. By treating certain allergies in their early stages, more serious complications can be avoided. People who know they are allergic can avoid the substances that are the cause of their allergy. A skin test can be performed to find out the allergic reaction. In this method, serum obtained from the blood of the allergic patient is injected into several sites in the skin of a non-allergic individual. This method is used when the patient himself has a poor diseased skin, which is not suitable for allergy test.

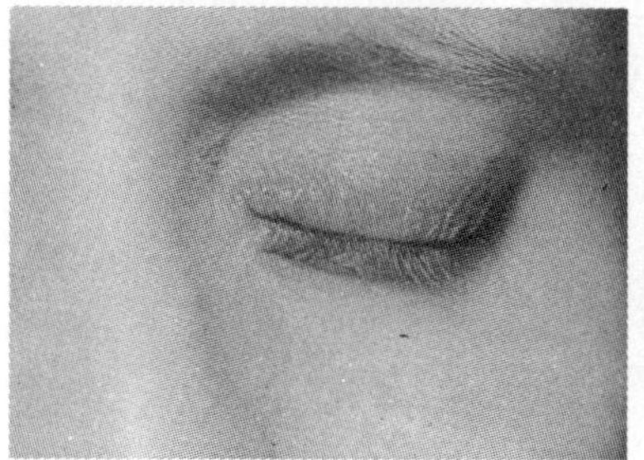

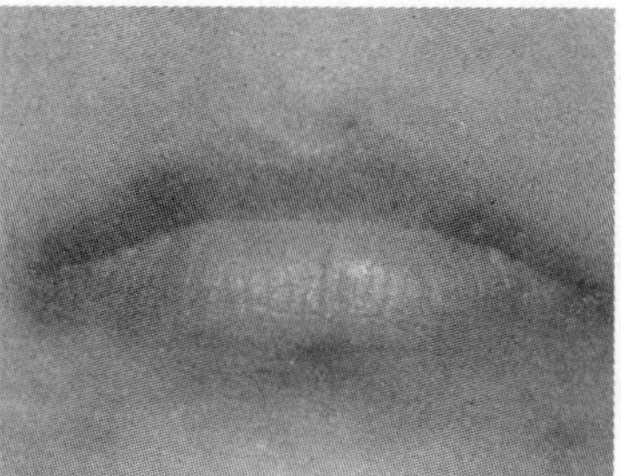

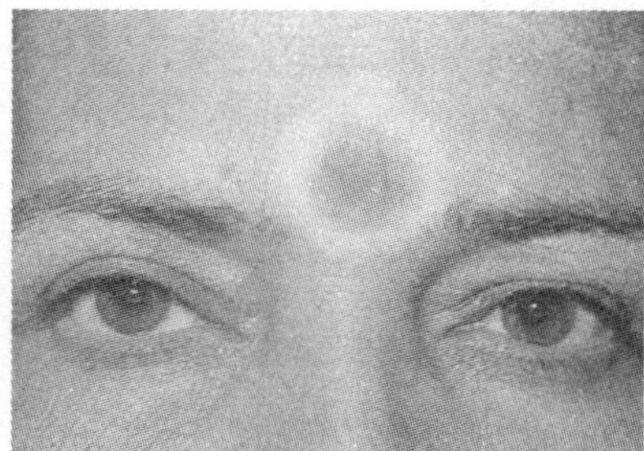

Eczema

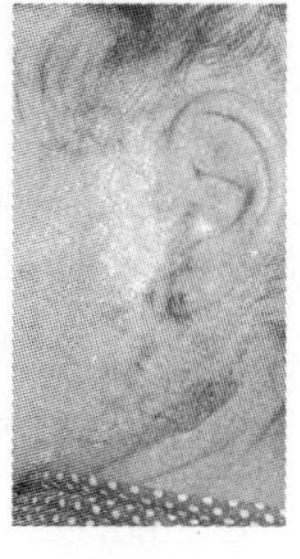

This is also known as **Dermatitis**—an inflammatory skin disorder in which the cuticle is fissured with a sticky, watery discharge. It starts with redness due to the dilated blood vessels. Fluid accumulates in the skin scabs and crusts. Apply a paste of *Babchi* mixed with mustard oil or leaves of *Mahua* (Indian Butter Tree) smeared with sesame oil on the affected skin. The infection accompanied with itching and pain is generally caused by the reaction of medicines or cosmetics.

Eczema—Dermatitis

Some do's and don'ts:

- **Relieve stress:** Stress can cause or contribute to flare-ups of eczema. Meditation can help a person with eczema release the stress.
- **Aromatherapy treatment:** A combination of the anti-inflammatory essential oils–German chamomile and high-alpine lavender—is considered one of the best therapies for soothing dermatitis. Put three to four drops of each oil in a base of ½ teaspoon of borage or evening primrose oil and apply the mixture on the affected skin.
- **Oatmeal bath:** Take an oatmeal bath as a soap substitute. Mix two cups of colloidal oatmeal (available at leading pharmacies) into a tub of lukewarm water.
- Topical creams, ointments and lotions containing cortisone are used to alleviate the itching and inflammation of eczema (dermatitis).
- Wear cotton clothes if suffering from eczema. Avoid acrylics.
- Calamine lotion is good for many types of rashes caused by eczema that ooze and may need to be dried out.
- Rapid change in air temperature is harmful for eczema patients. An air-conditioned room to a hot shower or a hot atmosphere can trigger itching.

Ringworm

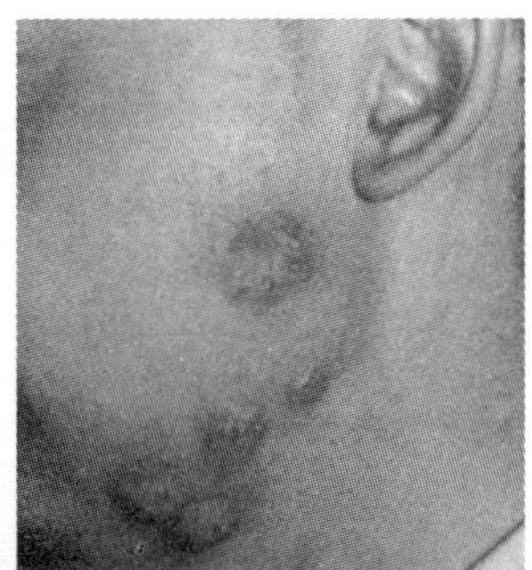

A fungal infection, harming the skin, in which round patches are formed on the body, especially between the legs, on the face, the neck, the back and on the buttocks. It is also known as *Tinea Corporis.* This malady is caused due to the inflammatory infection of the skin produced by certain moulds. Scratch the affected skin and apply borax mixed with lime juice. Apply the juice of marigold *(genda)* or basil *(tulsi)* leaves.

Freckles

Freckles are small, irregular, brownish, pigmented spots or scar (sometimes in round patches) generally caused due to excessive exposure to sun. The following treatment is suggested:

- Mix a few drops of lime juice to a tablespoon of milk cream and apply on the affected skin at night before going to bed.
- Pick up a vitamin E capsule, break it open and let the oil ooze out over the spot. Helps the wound heal.
- Eat a well-balanced diet containing protein and vitamins. Mineral zinc is of particular importance to heal freckles.
- Grind turmeric and sesame seeds in equal quantity and apply the paste on the skin.
- Mix yellow mustard in milk and apply the paste on the skin at night before sleep, wash thoroughly next morning.

Red veins

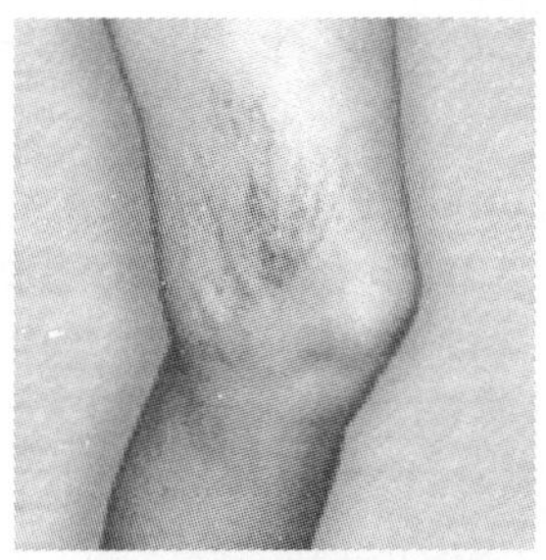

The skin becomes red and thin, blood vessels seem very near to the surface, usually caused due to sensitive, neglected or ill-treated skin. Apply some waxy cream, use moisturisers, avoid going out to the extremes of temperature and avoid rich, spicy foods as well as very hot drinks and alcohol.

Cracked skin and open pores

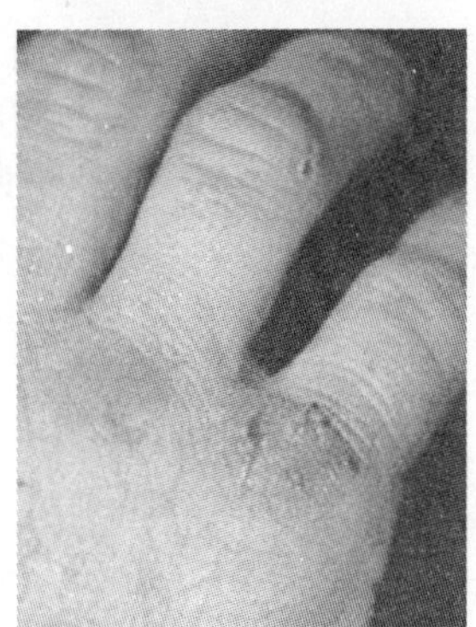

The lips get chapped, the skin of the hands get cracks, generally occurring due to cold with the onset of winter or defective functioning of the sebaceous glands. Rub a little castor oil or olive oil on the skin, apply hot milk cream on the cracked skin, use antibiotic cream and massage the affected skin at night. In case of open pores, the face looks unattractive and the skin gives the appearance of enlarged pores caused by over-active glands due to puberty. If you have a poor diet and/or an emotional disturbance, then use a face mask, twice a week. To make a face pack, mix 2 tablespoons of honey with ½ tbsp. of lime juice and 1 tbsp. of rose water. Another remedy is to apply a face mask. Mix cucumber juice with fuller's earth (*multani mitti*) or gramflour. Let it dry for ten minutes and then wash.

Red nose and prickly heat

Severe itching and burning are symptoms of red nose—(a common trouble with hearty eaters and drinkers and sudden change of temperature on delicate skin). Avoid sudden change of temperature and massage your nose up and down with rose water mixed with glycerine. Red pustules of the size of mustard grains appear on the body, especially on the chest, back and the abdomen due to profuse sweating during hot or rainy days and prickly heat. Apply green *henna* and leaves of *neem* ground in water on the affected skin. A pack of fuller's earth leaves a cooling effect on the skin. Avoid wearing heavy garments. Expose the affected area to fresh air and have a cold water bath twice in a day.

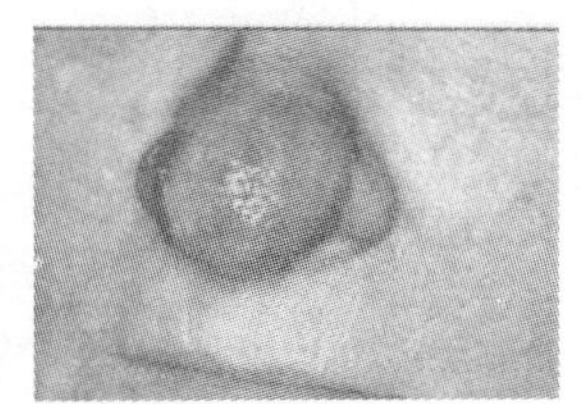

Muddy skin

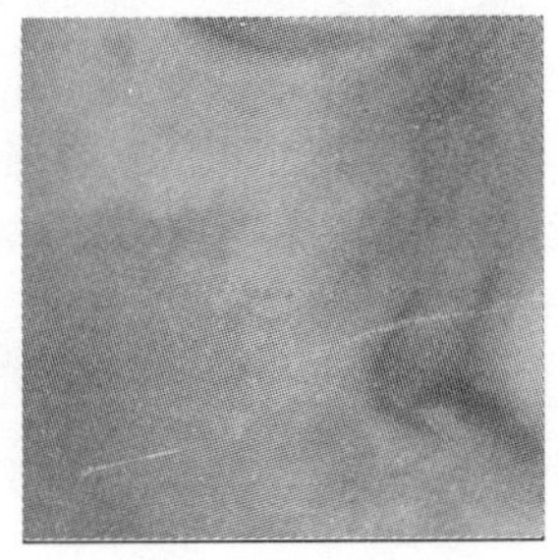

The skin loses its radiance due to over-tiredness and lack of sleep. As remedial measures, drink a glass of hot skimmed milk at night before going to bed, drink 4–6 glasses of cold water everyday between meals (not with the meals), take fresh fruits and green vegetables as much as you can, and have cold drinks and fruit juices without sugar.

Cold Sores (Virus—*Herpes simplex*)

Tiny white blisters appear in the corners of mouth and around the lips, generally seen in children. It is an infectious disease and sometimes, affects the genitalia due to sexual intercourse with some one from the opposite sex suffering from the disease. Herpes can be dangerous because of dehydration and the spread of infection to the hands and eyes. Some do's and don'ts to get rid of cold sores are as follows:

- ***Foods that must be avoided*:** If you are prone to oral herpes, you should not have foods that contain arginine such as nuts (almonds, cashews, peanuts and walnuts), seeds (sunflower and sesame), pork, milk and cheese.
- The acidophilus bacteria found in yoghurt helps counter the herpes virus.
- The cold compress of ice wrapped in a napkin or washcloth stops blisters and relieves pain. Keep it on your skin for 15–30 minutes.
- Minerals such as calcium and magnesium help keep the body's pH level alkaline, which is a necessary step in preventing cold sores.
- In case of recurrent attacks of herpes, have Acyclovir treatment with the consultation of your doctor.
- Do not keep your toothbrush in the bathroom. The moisture helps prolonging the life of the herpes virus on your toothbrush. Keep your toothbrush at a dry place.
- **Beta-Carotene:** This vitamin strengthens the mucous membranes of the mouth and hastens the healing of a cold sore. Vitamin E, a nutrient, also builds immunity and integrity of the epithelium and speeds up healing those with chronic problems.
- Use small tubes of toothpaste, usually toothpaste can transmit disease.
- Protect your cold sore by covering it with petroleum jelly. Use a fresh cotton swab when applying the jelly.
- Lemon balm ointment soothes cold sores.

Hypersensitive skin

This skin is prone to redness, blotchy and broken veins due to change in temperatures. Make-up causes swelling, blotches, irritation and reacts violently even on delicate skins causing allergies. Avoid extremes of temperature, cut out rich and spicy foods and stop taking liquor. Avoid very hot or cold water bath and use of soap.

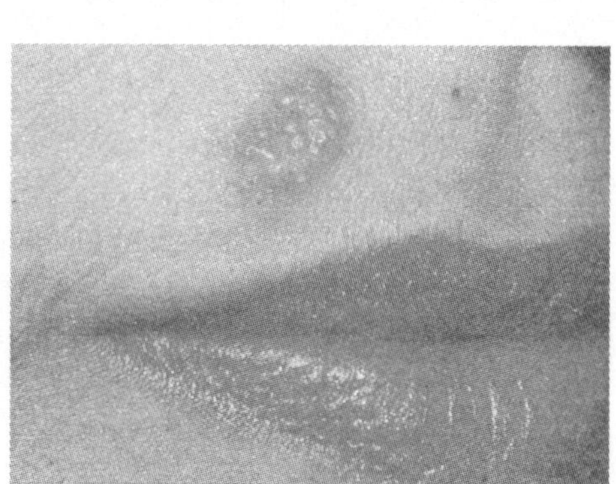

Birthmarks

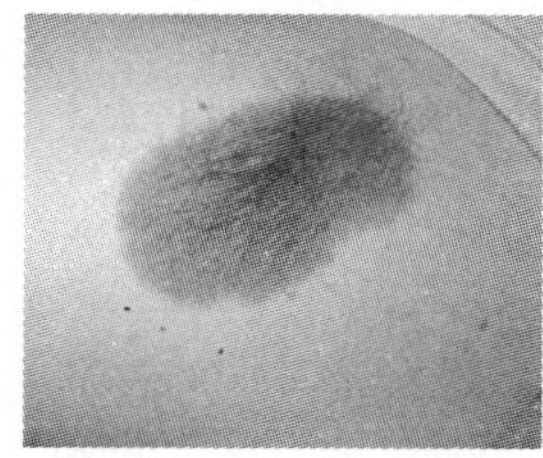

Caused by dark brown patches or fairly small moles by scratching the pimples or small-pox marks that disfigure the skin and leave a permanent scar. Remedial measures include treating the scars with carbon snow, ray treatment and cortisone injections. Minor scars can be eradicated by skin grafting or cosmetic surgery by a skin specialist. Strawberry marks can be removed by electric coagulation or by X-ray treatment or a peeling treatment.

Sunburn

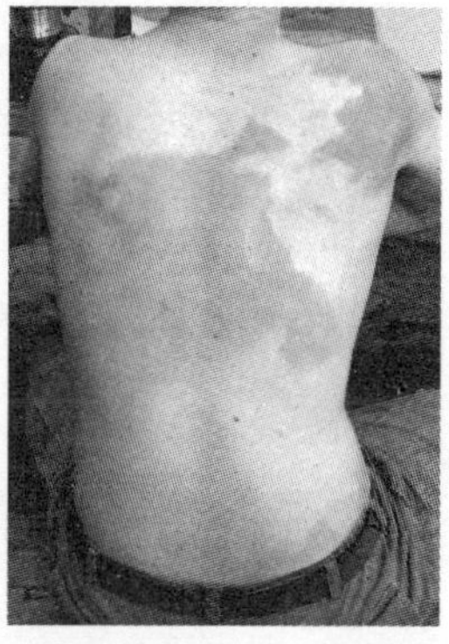

A severe sunburn is very bad for you. Consult a doctor immediately if you experience nausea, chills, fever, faintness, extensive blistering, general weakness, patches of purple discolouration, intense itching and if the burn seems to be spreading. Most sunburns are first-degree burns in which you have roasted your epidermis, the outer layer of the skin, and it is red, painful and hot. The second-degree burn involves the dermis or the underlying skin layer, which causes swelling, blisters, intense pain and perhaps nausea, chills and fever as the body tries to cope with the shock. In this case, you need to seek immediate medical care. Dryness of the skin due to dehydration causes scarring of the skin and it loses its complexion becoming dark, thick, leathery, wrinkled and patchy due to the adverse effect of the sun on the skin. The following treatment is recommended in case of sunburn:

- Drink at least 8–10 glasses of water a day in summer and 4–6 glasses a day in winter.
- There is no better remedy for minor burns (including to relieve pain, heat and redness) than aloe gel. For better treatment, get the gel directly from the leaves. Squish out the gel from the leaves and spread it on the burn. Leave for 3–5 minutes a day as much as your skin will absorb until the burn is healed. Essential oil, lavender, etc., when mixed to few drops of aloe gel and spread on the burned skin and several inches on the surrounding area, encourages new skin development in that area.
- Yoghurt is very cooling and a natural moisturiser, when applied liberally to the burned skin for 10–15 minutes. Repeat this three to four times a day.
- Aspirin can help relieve the pain, itching and swelling due to sunburn. Consult a doctor, who will usually recommend two tablets every four hours.
- Apply soothing compresses following a burn when the skin is inflamed. Use plain water to which a few ice cubes are added. Dip a cloth into the liquid and place it over the burn. Skimmed milk, too, is very soothing due to its nutrient value. Use milk instead of water for better results. Moisten a cloth with witch-hazel and apply on the affected skin for temporary relief.

- Add soothing, anti-inflammatory ingredients to a bath and soak for 10-20 minutes twice a day, until the sunburn is gone. Add a cup of black tea (anti-inflammatory tannins) and one cup of apple-cider vinegar (a time-tested, soothing sunburn remedy) to the bath water (neither too cold nor too hot) and soak. For excellent results, add 6-7 drops of lavender in the bath water.
- Apply a sun-tan lotion or cream before going out. Apply a sunscreen about 30 minutes before going out. Do not forget to protect your lips, hands, ears and the back of your neck. Reapply as necessary after swimming or perspiring heavily. Take extra care between 11.00 a.m. and 4.00 p.m. when the sun is at its hottest.
- If you develop blisters, you have a pretty bad burn. For skin that is blistering, you must seek medical advice. Antioxidant vitamins will help the skin heal more rapidly from sunburn. The sun causes oxidative damage to the skin cells, and the antioxidants speed up recovery. Continue the following doses daily for a week in consultation with your doctor.

  Vitamin A : 10,000 IU

  Vitamin C : 1,000 milligrams

  Vitamin E : 400 IU

Boils and Pustules

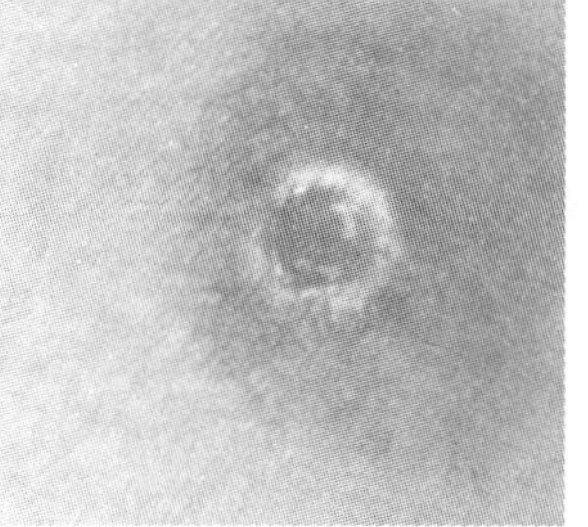

Boils—red, small, painful nodules that start oozing pus and leave tiny scars are a bacterial infection of a sweat gland or hair follicle, and usually found on the face, in the armpit, on groin, neck, knees, elbows and buttocks. When blocked by dead skin cells and other debris, which creates pus along with redness, swelling and pain, are called pustules. Recurrent boils are caused by gastro-intestinal bacteria, which enter the blood stream and promote a skin infection. Never lance or press a boil to open it as this can spread the infection and cause scarring. The following tips help to stop infection:

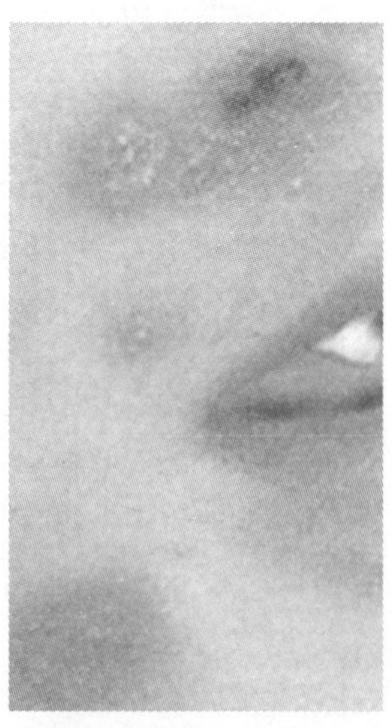

- The treatment should be done by a qualified dermatologist, which may include antibiotics, draining the pustule or a steroid injection.
- In Ayurveda, the ancient natural healing system, boils are seen as a 'pitta' disorder—an excess of fire and heat. Turmeric is a cooling herb, helps to reduce inflammation and prevent recurrences. Make turmeric paste and apply on the boil three times a day until it is cured. To make a paste, combine and blend—450 milligrams turmeric powder, 1 teaspoon of Epsom salt and a baked onion. Spread the paste on a cloth bandage, place over the boil and leave the poultice on overnight.

- Treat the boil with just hot compresses, followed by cold compresses (ice-cold water compress) to draw out the pus.
- Apply a paste of *neem* tree bark on the boil, three times a day.
- Smear a leaf of *peepal* tree with warm *ghee* and apply as a bandage over the boil.
- Apply a warm washcloth compress over the boil changing after every three to four hours as below:
    * A heated slice of tomato.
    * A raw onion slice.
    * Mashed garlic.
    * Leaves of cabbage.
    * A bag of black tea

Blackheads, acne and wrinkles

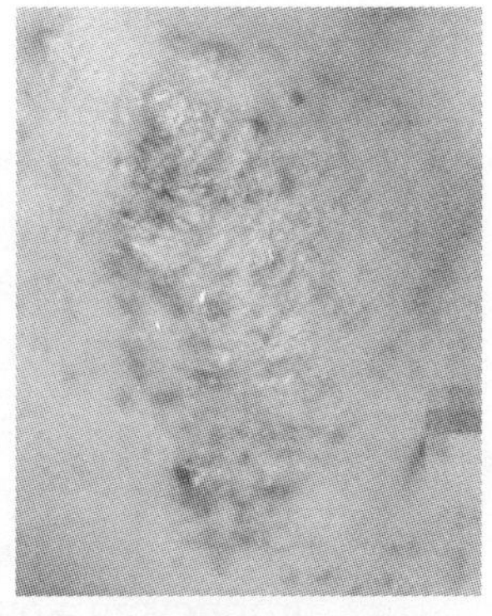

Small pimples on the skin which get inflamed, ooze pus and are caused due to over-active skin oozing grease. Remedial cures include washing the skin, three times a day with a medicated soap, if the skin is greasy. Have a balanced diet. Avoid taking fried foods, chocolates, pastries, spices and aerated drinks. Unclog skin pores by steaming and applying a face pack. Do not scratch pimples. Wrinkles give an old look to a young person. It is caused by loosening of the skin tissues and muscles, dryness of the skin, irritation, annoyance, anger and mental tension. To delay ageing, the measures to counter wrinkles are facial massage, use of a cream containing vitamin C, facial exercises, using a good moisturising cream, having a protein-rich diet and avoiding bright sun rays.

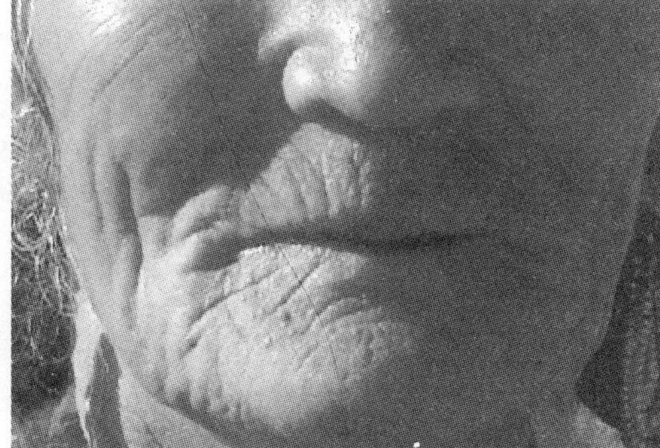

Wrinkles: Wrinkled skin is not a life-threatening problem like that of grey hair. Grey hair can, however, be touched up with a dye. But you cannot iron out wrinkles. Wrinkles can cause premature ageing.

Here is a home recipe to fight wrinkles:

Mix in a bowl 1 teaspoon of fuller's earth, 1 teaspoon of oatmeal or oat flour, 1 teaspoon avocado or olive oil, ½ tablespoon powdered milk, 2 teaspoons of honey and enough water to make a paste. Add to it, two to three drops of essential oil of frankincense.

Apply the pack to your face evenly avoiding the area around eyes. Leave for 10 minutes while you lie down with your feet slightly elevated. Cover your eyes with an eye pad moistened with rose water. When the pack is dry, rinse with lukewarm water and follow with a cool water splash. Use this pack two to three times a month.

Steps to eradicate wrinkles:

- Avoid excess exposure to sun. The main reason that skin wrinkles is that it loses moisture as the components in our skin that have the ability to hold moisture decrease with age. Spray your face with fine mist of water three times a day, which can help soften and plump the surface of dried, wrinkled skin, reducing the fine lines.
- Aromatherapy delays ageing. Mix one drop each of essential oil of the herbs neroli, primrose or borage. Put the mixture on a cotton pad and wipe your face with it after your cleansing routine. This toner firms sagging skin. These essential oils are rich in gamma-linolenic acid (GLA)—one of the fatty acids involved in collagen production.
- Massage can help reduce lines on your forehead. Use sesame or almond oil for massage. Mix to it two drops each of sandalwood and geranium essential oils and one drop each of lemon and cardamom oil. Gently massage with your fingers to nourish, soothe and energise the skin.
- Avoid exposure to sunlight, which breaks down the collagen and elastin in your skin causing wrinkles.
- Do not smoke, since cigarette smoking deprives your skin of oxygen and nutrients. Smoking can cause lines around the corners of your mouth and vertical lines in your upper lip.
- Avoid using soap, choose cleansing lotions instead of soap. Soaps foam up and draw out natural oils from the skin and age it prematurely.
- Limit coffee and alcohol to one cup or one drink a day. The excess quantity may reduce the quantity of water and nutrients in your body and wrinkle the skin.
- Include foods such as vegetables, fruits, grains, beans, nuts, seeds and low-fat dairy products in your diet.
- Make sure you get enough vitamin D if you stay away of the sun. Sunlight provides us with essential vitamin D. You can also get vitamin D-enriched milk or a multivitamin tablet.
- Keep pillows away from your face. Watch out for sleep wrinkles, which are caused by pressing your face into the pillow at night. Learn to sleep on your back or find a position where your face is not pressing the pillow.
- Exercise regularly for healthier, wrinkle-free skin and avoid ageing.
- Eat right. Vitamins and minerals are important to maintain a youthful skin. Among the most important vitamins include vitamin A and C (found in fresh fruits and vegetables), vitamin B-complex (found in chicken, eggs, whole wheat and milk). Best foods for healthy skin are green leafy vegetables, carrots and fresh fruits.
- Use a moisturiser to hide some of the smaller wrinkles. Dampen the skin before applying a moisturiser.
- Live with less stress. Remember, a stressful lifestyle enhances wrinkles and premature ageing.

Rhinoplasty (Deformed nose)

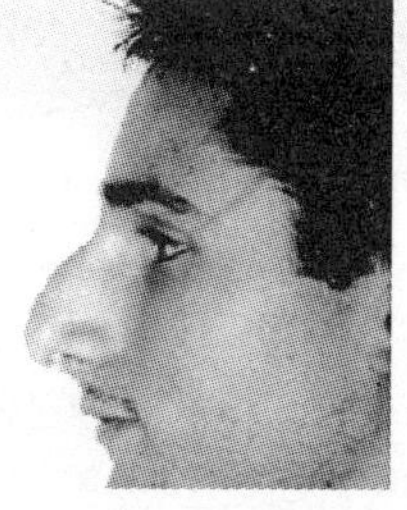

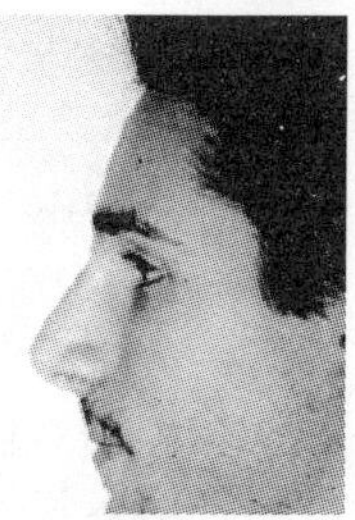

A hump nose deformity in which the skin of upper part of the nose becomes free from the underlying the bone and cartilage giving a saddle nose look. Surgery is done to carve the hump and reduce deformity. The steps include removal of the hump, nasal infracture, elevation of the tip of the nose and trimming of the lower part.

Moles and warts

Warts are viruses that can grow anywhere on the surface of the body. These are benign skin tumours that can occur singly or in large packs on the body. Warts should be diagnosed accurately and treated appropriately. In genital area, warts can be sexually transmitted and may cause cervical cancer. Once the warts are diagnosed, they should be removed immediately rather than waiting until they spread and enlarge and become difficult to eliminate at later stage. Warts—pink, brown and black, hairy or hairless swellings (called neo-plasins), usually occur on the face, fingers and the trunk. They usually multiply and grow into the dermis. Treat your wart with the following methods:

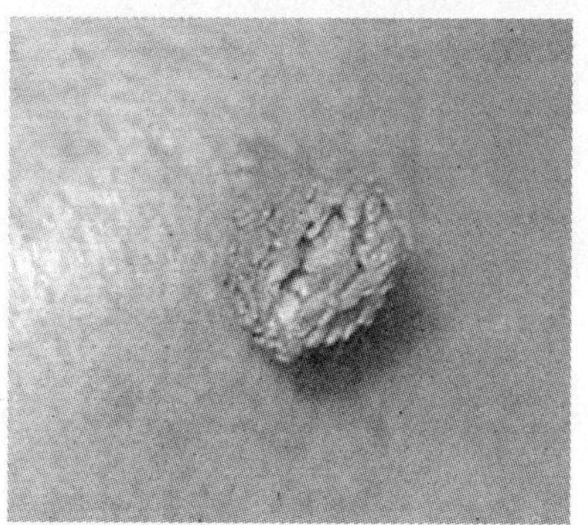

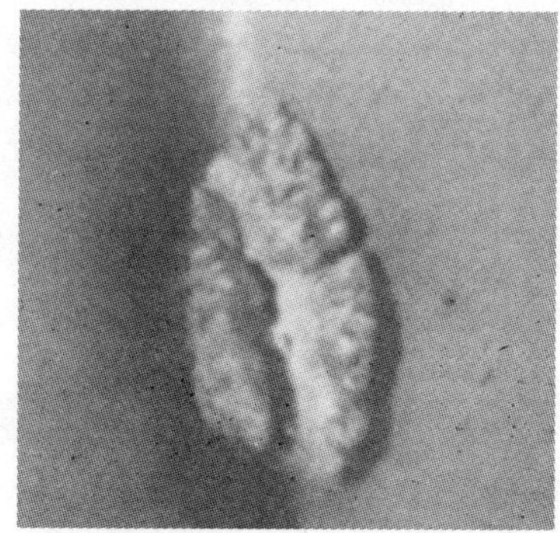

- Warts are easily removed by cryosurgery or freezing with liquid nitrogen and electro-cautery (a procedure that burns the wart off with an electrified surgical tool).
- Garlic oil is a traditional remedy for warts. Swab the oil on the wart or on a bandage applied to the wart.
- Patients with warts should take a daily multivitamin/mineral supplement that includes minimum 200 micrograms of selenium (a strong anti-viral nutrient), 10,000 IU of vitamin A, 500 milligrams of vitamin C, 400 IU of vitamin E and 15 milligrams of zinc.
- Apply a peeling agent daily (4% sulphur calamine lotion or Retino A cream available with any chemist shop). Treatment should be done strictly as per the doctor's prescription.
- Mind-body technique such as self-hypnosis is very effective for healing warts. To practice this, sit comfortably on a chair relaxing the body with deep breaths. Form a mental picture of a patch of snow over your wart daily for five minutes. Your wart starts melting.

- Remember, warts are caused by a virus. It exists in the air and you pick it up as in viral infection. Wart virus thrives in a very moist environment.
- Warts spread quickly. Try not to touch it with your hand.
- Apply vitamin E oil, clove oil, aloe vera juice, milkweed juice and milky juice of unripe figs directly to the wart.
- Take garlic capsules or tablets after consulting your doctor.
- Soak lemon slices in apple cider with a little salt for two weeks; then rub the lemon slices on the wart.
- Tape the inner side of a banana skin to a planter wart.
- Rub wart with a piece of a raw potato.

Planter wart: A planter wart is a wart on the bottom of your feet. The virus produces more viruses and virus-carrying cells. Putting garlic directly on a planter wart can help get rid of it. Mash a clove of garlic into pulp, put the pulp directly on the wart at night, cover it with a small adhesive bandage, remove bandage in the morning and clean the area. If the planter wart is painful and bleeds, you should have it removed. The most effective method of removal of a planter wart is application of liquid nitrogen, which freezes and kills the wart so that it falls off. Another method for the removal of planter wart is a surgical laser. Astragalus is one of the best herbs for strengthening the immune system and preventing the occurrence of planter warts.

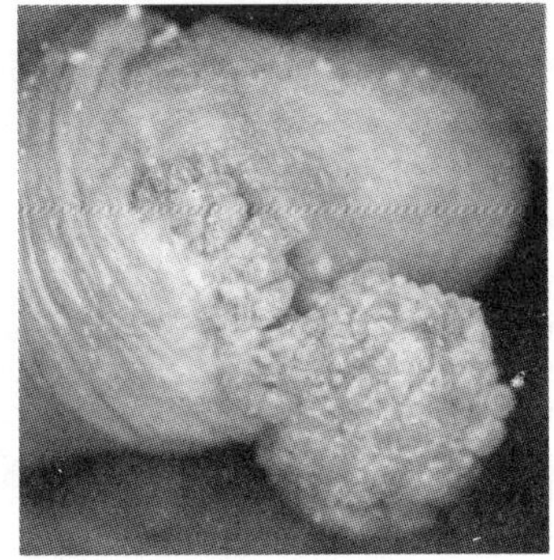

Leucoderma (white patches)

Painless white spots or patches on the body, which expand if not treated, are caused due to loss of pigmentation in the skin. To prevent the spread of leucoderma, protect from exposure to excessive heat, have salt-free diet and apply *chandan* pack on the patches. Soak the seeds of *Babchi* in ginger juice for 72 hours, remove their husk, dry and powder, and apply it on the patches.

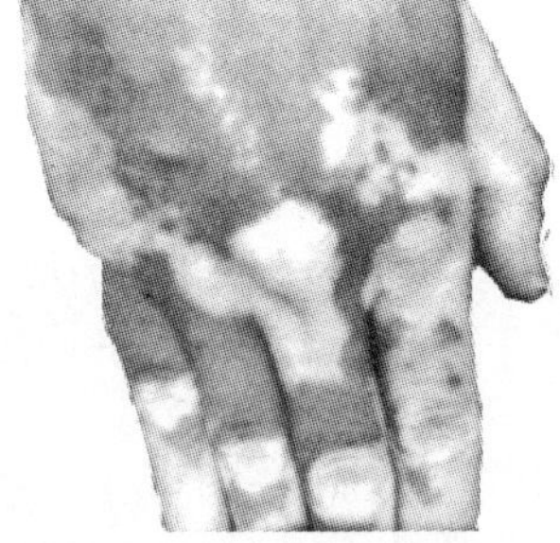

Leucoderma is curable; it is not a contagious disease. Generally, an imbalance of melanin in the body results in the appearance of white patches. Darker skins have more patches because such skins carry more melanin. It is clarified that these white patches are not congenital nor hereditary. Children are not affected if the mother suffers from leucoderma. It is untrue that women suffering from this disease cannot enjoy marital pleasure.

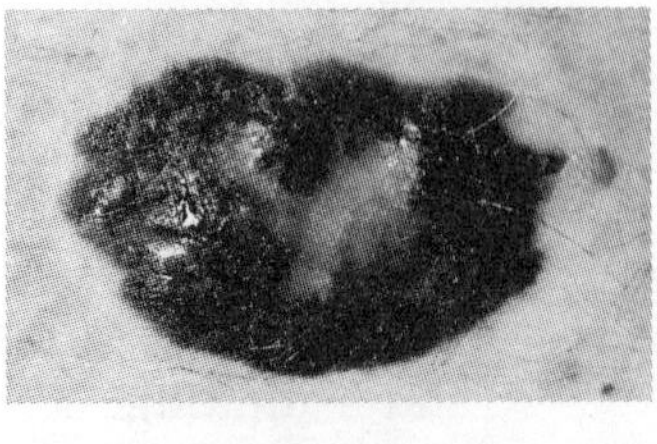

Skin cancers (Keratoses)

Scaly patches on the scalp, face and back of the hands develop in elderly persons usually on areas exposed to sun or due to X-ray treatment and exposure to toxic chemicals. Treatment should be done by radio-therapy, surgery and cryotherapy in which liquid nitrogen can be used to kill the cancer cells by freezing.

Leprosy

The skin starts whitening and slowly massive round lumps are formed on it. The disease affects the eyes, leading to blindness. Fingers fall off at the joints and the skin over the palms starts rotting. This is an infectious disease. Remedies include a daily massage with *neem* soap or application *neem* oil on the affected area. Boil leaves of *neem* and *amaltas* and take a bath in the water. Take a salt-free diet and avoid constipation.

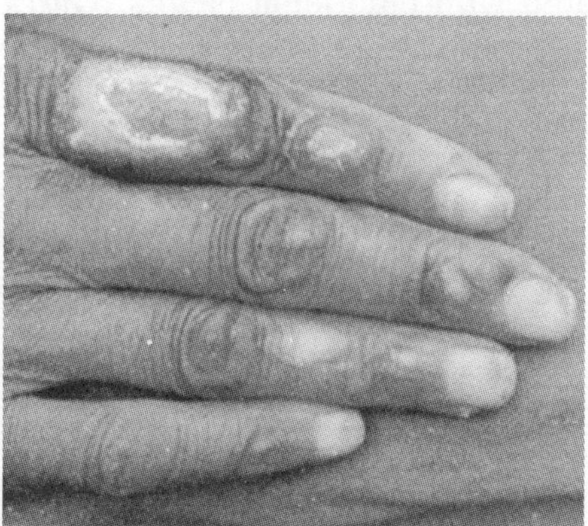

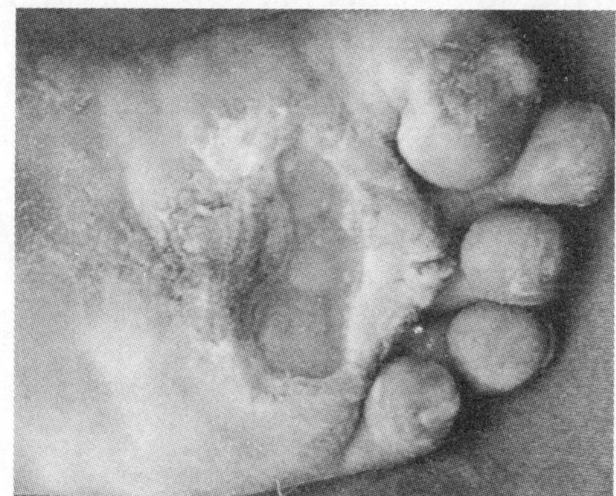

Skin tumour

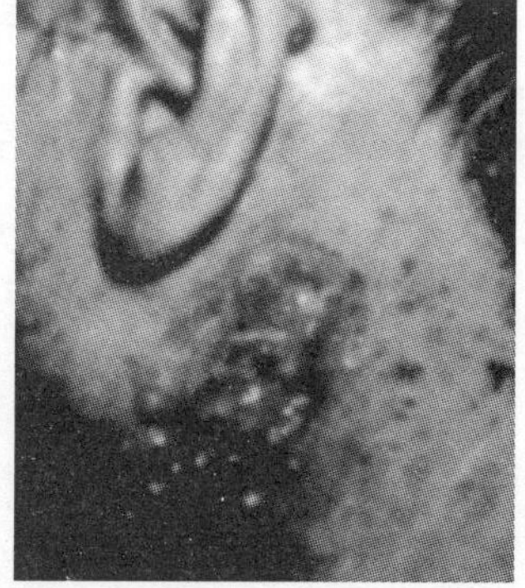

Seborrhoeic warts appear on the skin and are caused by excessive exposure to sun's rays. If not treated in time, it leads to skin cancer. It can be only removed surgically.

Crow's feet

Lines and wrinkles appear on the face. The skin hangs in folds and wrinkles appear around the eyes causing ageing. Apply sesame or coconut oil over the face and neck before sleep. Remember that anger and irritation add to the lines of age on the face. Douche with warm and then cold water alternatively. Avoid rubbing the skin with towel but massage lightly.

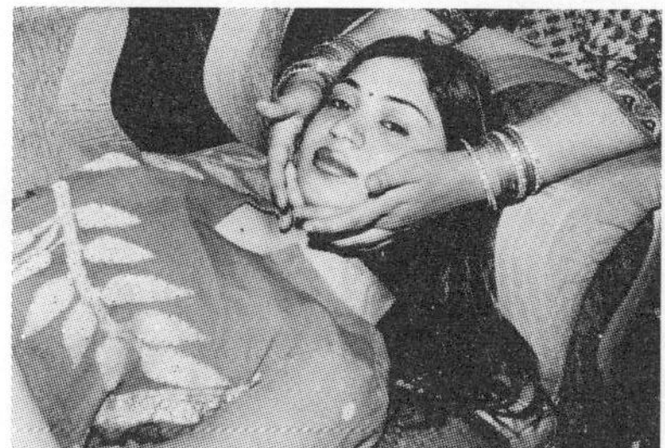

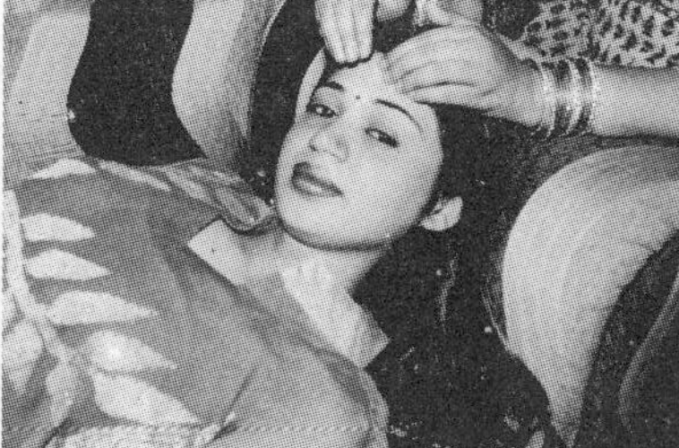

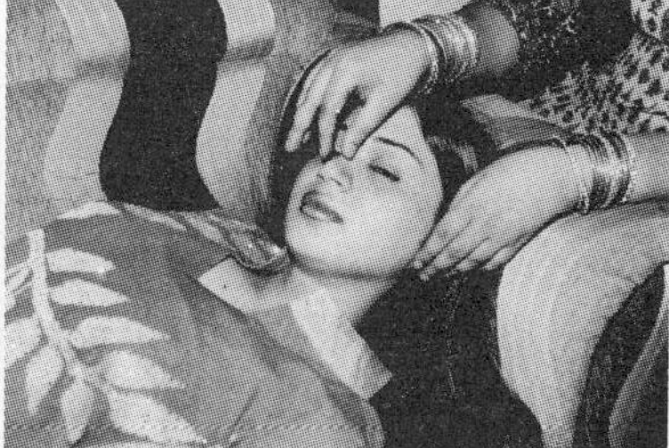

Urticaria (Hives)

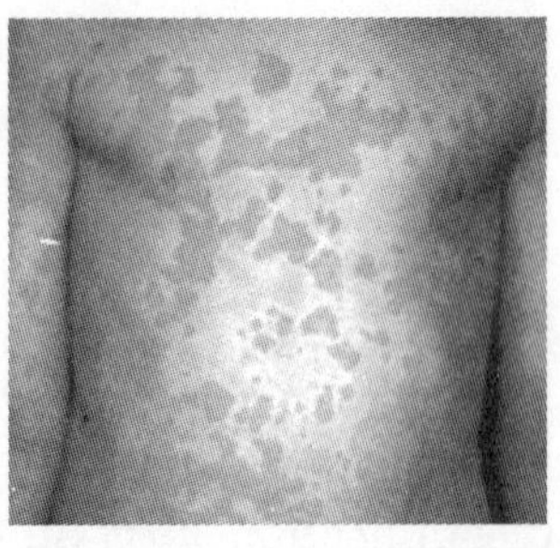

A swollen area of the skin surrounded by a red wheal and generally known as *nettle rash.* Equal quantity of alum and red ochre *(geru)* should be ground together and the powder rubbed on the wheals. In case of severe itching, mix 3 parts of rose water and 2 parts of vinegar and apply.

Psoriasis *(Eka Kushta)*

A scaly eruption of the skin. Red patches develop covered by scale, which can be itchy. It is caused due to impurities in the blood associated with emotional factors. *Guggulu Tiktaka Ghrita* is given internally to improve digestion and remove impurities from the blood. Spicy food, curds and salt should be avoided. One may use a little rock salt. *Neem* leaves (ground) applied on the area will be helpful.

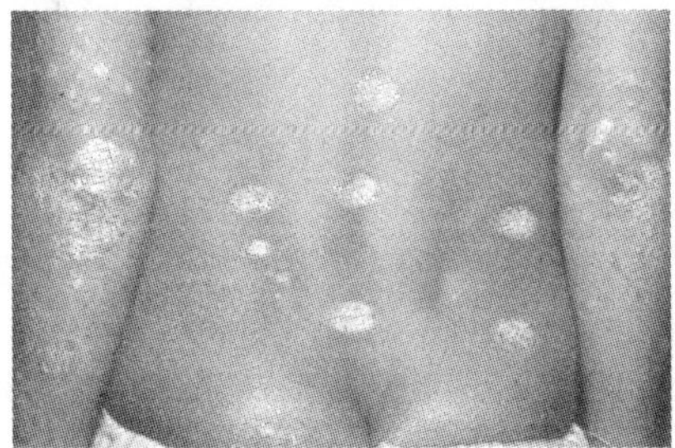

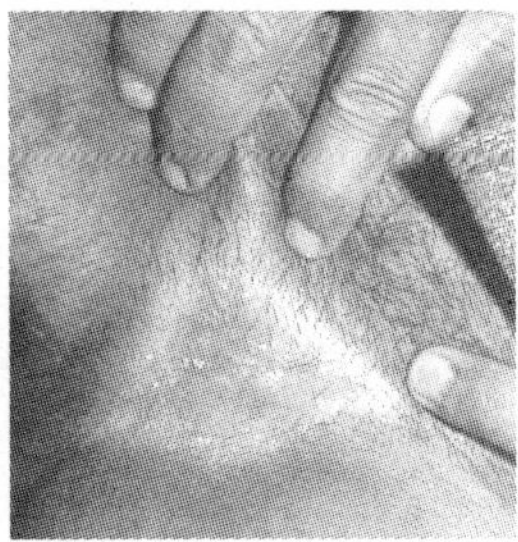

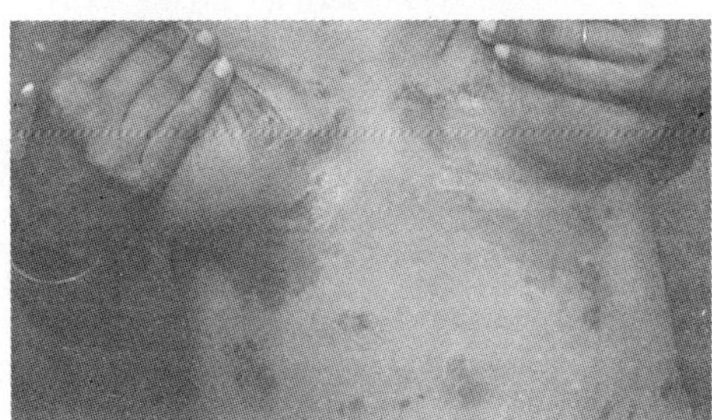

Remedies to treat Psoriasis: Psoriasis is a serious disease, often severe condition requires professional care. It is difficult to diagnose this disease and wrong medication leaves side-effects. Vitamin D or vitamin A based-ointments generally suggested to treat psoriasis can sometimes have long-term side-effects.

- Water is the best internal cleanser to expel toxins from the body. Psoriasis patients should drink six to eight glasses of water everyday.
- Rub castor oil on thick skin or a mixture of olive oil and peanut oil in equal quantity to moisturise the thinner lesions.
- Exercise is a vital part of the regimen for clearing psoriasis. It stimulates the internal structures of the body, increases circulation, activates the glands, oxygenates the blood, opens the skin pores and filters the blood through the liver and kidneys. A daily aerobic activity such as walking, swimming, cycling and playing tennis or badminton for 30-40 minutes is helpful.
- Bathing (body cleansing) begins to throw off accumulated toxins. In case of increased burning and itching, a bath in lukewarm water to which one cup of apple cider and one cup rolled oats is added, is quite helpful.
- ***Food you must eat or avoid:*** Stay away from white potatoes, peppers and tomatoes, processed foods, food prepared with coconut oil or palm oil, excess sweets, sodas, candy, pastries and fried food. Avoid smoking, since tobacco is a nightshade. However,

the diet for a psoriasis patient should be 70-80% fruits and vegetables. Take leafy green salads, grains, poultry, fish and low-fat, low-sodium dairy products.

- Get a small UVB sunlamp to treat patches of psoriasis.
- Sunbathing cures psoriasis. It gets worse in winter or in a humid climate.
- Weight loss helps people with psoriasis.
- Stress can trigger psoriasis.

Whitlow

An infection of the soft pad at the tip of the finger or thumb, tender to touch with pus formation. One part of *isphgula* should be steeped in four parts of vinegar and applied to the spot. The inflammation is likely to resolve in 2-3 days. Once the pus has been ejected, the *neem* leaves should be made into a poultice and bound over the affected site.

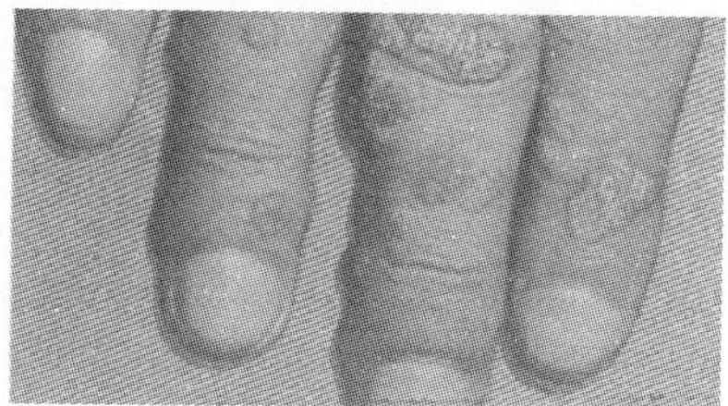

Acne Vulgaris: Prevention or cure

A common inflammatory cosmetic disease of the skin, mostly affecting the face, the upper part of the chest and the back. The exact cause is not known. It is believed to be due to seborrhoea and hormonal disturbances during adolescence. It mostly affects the teenagers. Acne is more common and severe in boys than girls. The predisposing factors include disorders of the digestive tract, hypovitaminosis of Vitamins A, E & B, Folic and Nicotinic acids, anaemia, malnutrition, infection, the character of diet and metabolism, overeating, excessive use of cosmetics, excessive medication and hereditary influences. Some clinical features of acne are mild soreness, itching or pain, papules or pustules, ectatic pores, acne cysts and scarring.

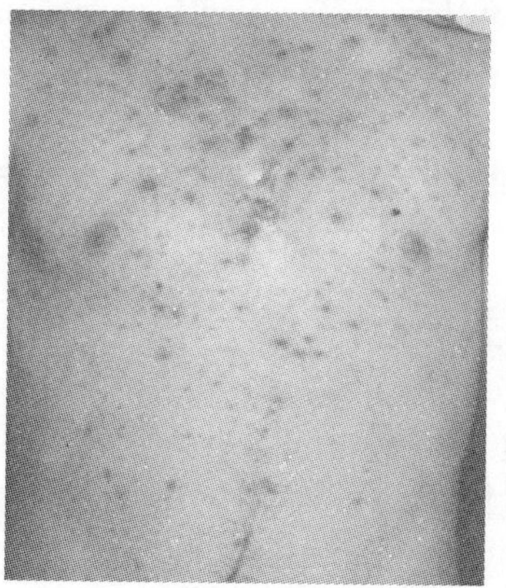

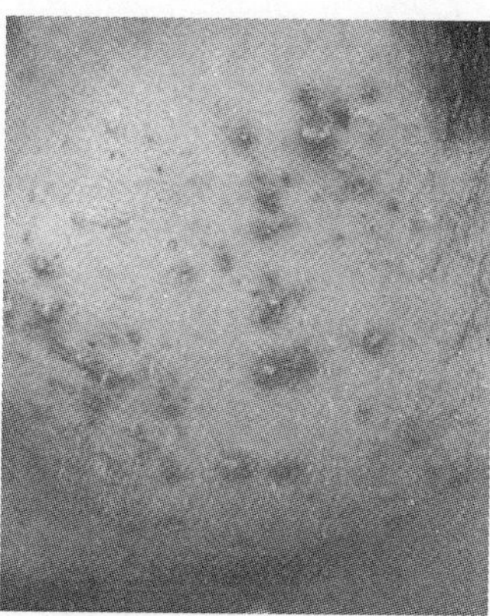

To Treat Acne

Education of the patient is essential not only to produce an acceptable cosmetic result while the condition is active, but also to prevent permanent scarring. Drink at least 8-10 glasses of water a day. Your diet should consist of more fruits, salads and should be easily digestible. Take citrus fruits. Avoid oily, spicy or fried food and chocolates. Eliminate medication. Avoid exposure to oil and grease and avoid cosmetics. Treat anaemia, malnutrition, infection and gastro-intestinal tract disorders. Wash the face 4-5 times a day. Regular *Yogasanas* and breathing exercises should be done to regulate the hormonal system. Face should be steamed with water to which *neem* leaves should be added. Simple exposure to late evening sunlight is often beneficial. Exposure to green and blue rays in the morning and evening help a lot. Splash the face with ice-cold water frequently. Apply *neem* paste on the acne skin frequently. Wash the face with lukewarm water and a face wash before sleep. Freshly prepared turmeric and sandalwood paste should be applied twice a day. Never break or squeeze the pustules, else they will become septic and leave permanent scars. During the pre-teen years, the skin maintains its natural beauty.

Herpes simplex

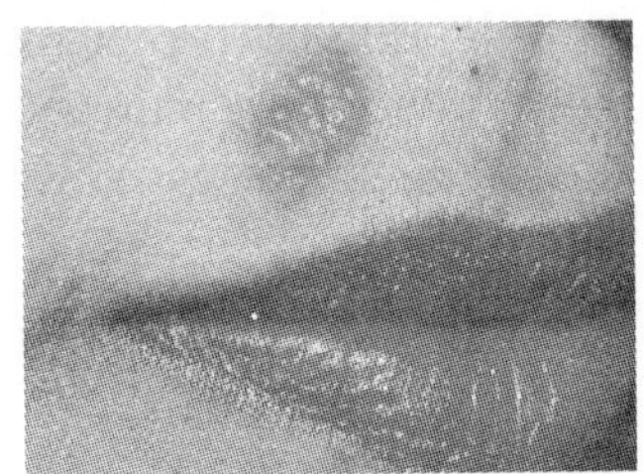

The attack of *Herpes* is usually severe. The lesions consist of multiple small vesicles or superficial ulcers on the upper lips and on the face in women and on the glans, penis and shaft of the penis in men. If the attack is mild, the lesions tend to heal in a week or two. However, if the infection is severe, consult a doctor (usually an antibiotic treatment is recommended).

Herpes zoster

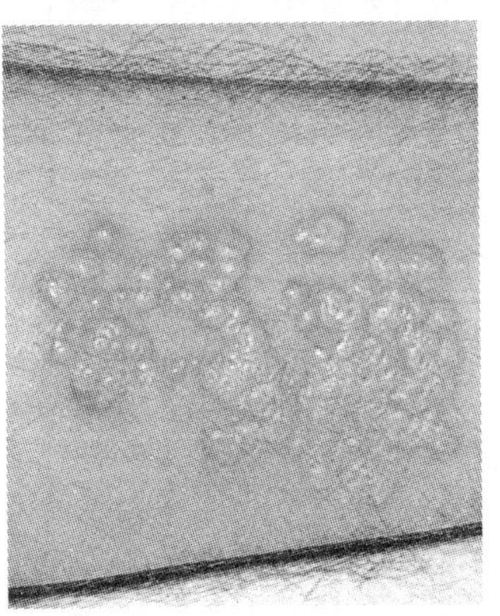

Is a virus infection commonly called *Blisters,* which usually appears on the genital areas, thighs and buttocks. The group of little blisters are painful, tender and highly infectious and burst in the meantime. Herpes zoster is caused by the same virus as that of the *Chicken pox*, usually caught by having sex with someone who has herpes (in case of Genital herpes), when a group of little blisters appear on the genital area. Soothe these blisters with essential oils of lemon, geranium, chamomile or lavender. The essential oils may be diluted in a base oil and rubbed on to the rash.

Herpes zoster (shingles) is a rashy infection caused by the Varicella zoster virus. It is a variety of the virus that causes oral and genital herpes and weakens the immune system, which later on causes shingles. Shingles is a painful but relatively harmless infection that can be treated with medications or home remedies. For those over the age 70, the pain of shingles never leaves a condition called post-herpetic neuralgia. If you have shingles blisters anywhere on or near the head (often meaning that you have AIDS, cancer or any other immune weakening disease) consult a doctor immediately. Also contact your doctor if you have difficulty in eating or drinking during an attack of shingles. Remember, internal blisters can be very serious. Acupuncture treatment helps relieve pain during an outbreak. There are several naturopathic home remedies to cure shingles:

- Activated charcoal draws the herpes virus out of the skin, quickly drying and healing blisters. Make a paste by mixing equal quantity of activated charcoal and cornstarch or ground flaxseed. Apply the paste on blisters with a piece of muslin. Leave the paste for at least 12 hours, then wash it off. Keep reapplying the paste until blisters are completely dry.

- A gel of hydrogen peroxide contains high levels of oxygen, which kills viruses.
- Capsaicin cream is an outstanding treatment for post-herpetic neuralgia–a condition that usually occurs in people over the age of 70.
- Vitamins and minerals contribute to the strength of the immune system. Doctors recommend high-potency multivitamin/mineral supplement if you have bout of shingles. Consult a doctor for suitable treatment. Vitamin C is the most important for healthy immune functioning (Recommended dose 2,000 mg. twice a day).
- Alpha-lipoic acid has powerful antioxidant properties, which helps prevent shingles outbreaks (consult a doctor for treatment).
- Amino acid lysine can help decrease the recurrence of shingles. Consult a doctor before treatment.
- Apply a wet dressing to eruptions. Take a washcloth or towel, dip it in cold water, squeeze it out and apply on the affected area.
- Heat is harmful in case of shingle blisters. Avoid anything that will make your blistered skin hotter.
- Use an antibiotic ointment strictly as per your doctor's advice.

Prickly heat

Red pustules the size of mustard grains appear on the body, especially on the chest, back and the abdomen. These are caused due to profuse sweating during hot and rainy season. Apply green *henna* ground in water on the affected area of the skin. Grind leaves of *neem* in water and apply on the affected skin. These are very effective treatments for *Prickly heat.*

Epidermolysis bullosa on knees and feet

This disorder is characterised by a tendency to develop blisters, ulcers, crusts and scars appearing on the knees and feet with the loss of nails many times. The disorder is seen between the epidermal layers by degeneration of the prickle and the basal cells. Application of vitamin E is beneficial.

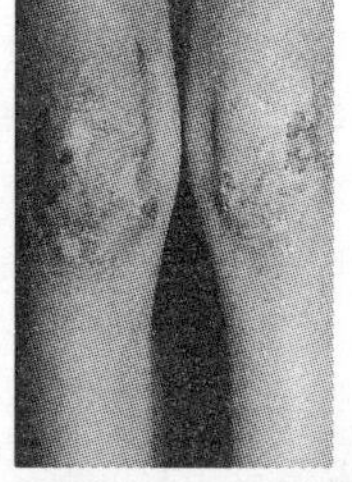

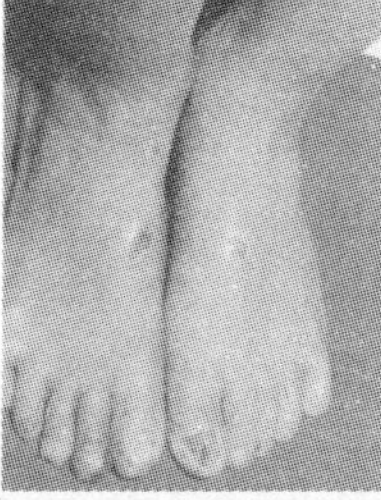

Ichthyosis vulgaris

A common hereditary disorder in which large brownish angulated scales appear on the body, especially on the legs (not on the face). The patient has a problem accompanied by papules over shoulders and buttocks. The lesions worsen in winter. Apply 40% urea dissolved in equal quantity of glycerine and water twice a day. Systematic usage of antibiotics is recommended.

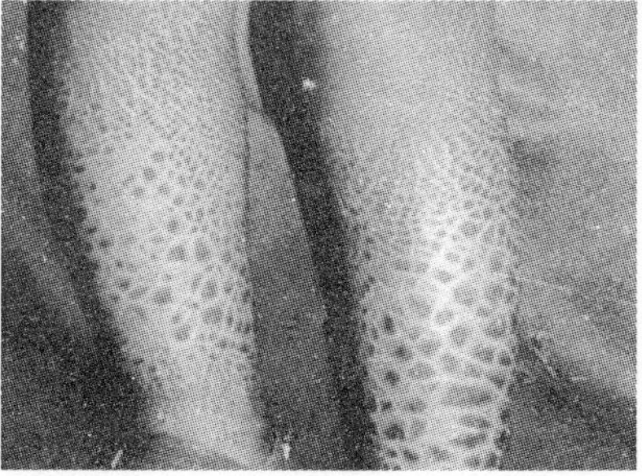

Pharynoderma

Deficiency of vitamin A or essential fatty acids lead to *Pharynoderma* in which hard keratonic follicular papules appear on the body, on the elbow, knees or the buttocks. *Night blindness, Bitot's spots and dryness of the skin* may also be associated. Local application of 10-40% urea cream along with intake of vitamin A can make the lesions disappear in due course.

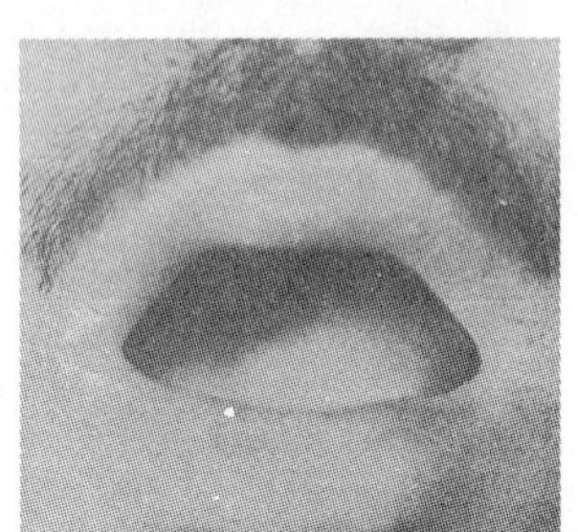

Angular stomatitis

A disorder caused by the deficiency of vitamin B complex causes a growth with a fissure at the angle of the mouth.

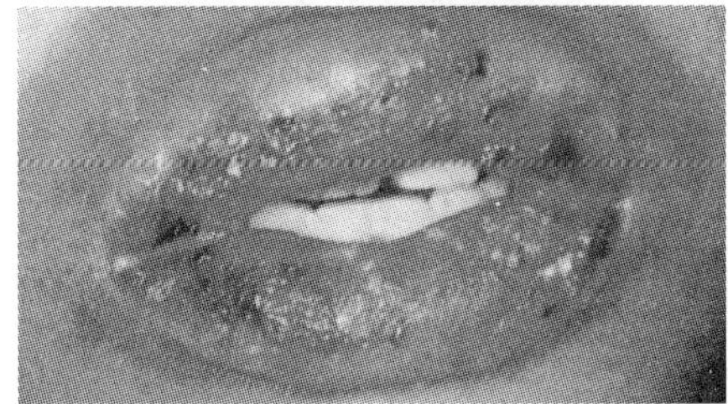

Cheilitis

Redness, scaling and swelling appear on both the lips in this condition.

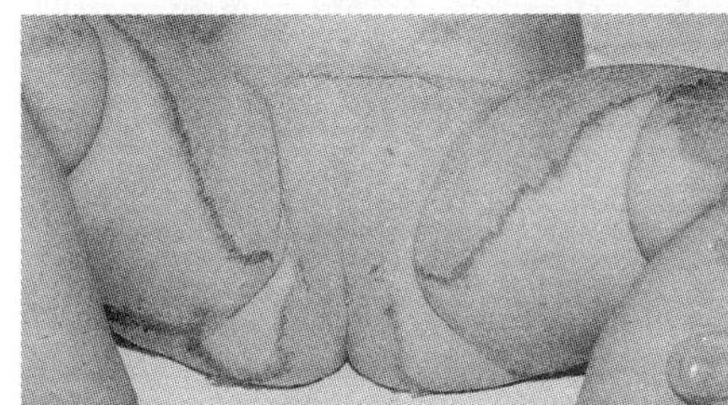

Acro-dermatitis Enteropathica

Deficiency of zinc in the mother's milk or an artificial feed usually in infants or in adults causes this disease following the gastro-intestinal tract. The trouble leads to vesiculation and ulceration around the nose, mouth, anal opening and genitalia.

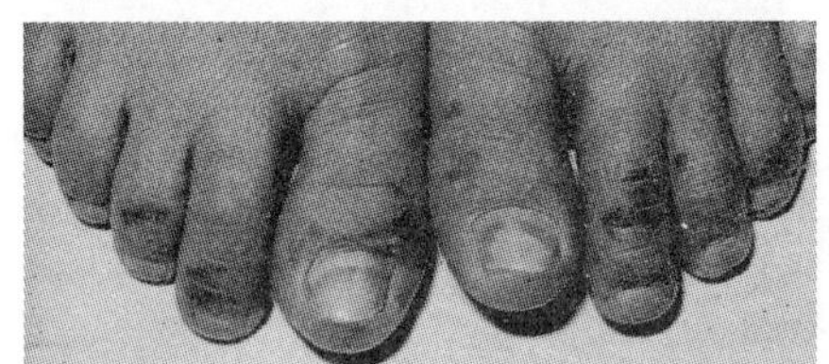

Chilblains

This condition causes lesions consisting of pain, brownish-black discolouration on toes and fingers which generally dies on exposure to cold. The treatment includes protection from cold and use of vasodilators during winter. The doctor usually recommends antibiotic treatment.

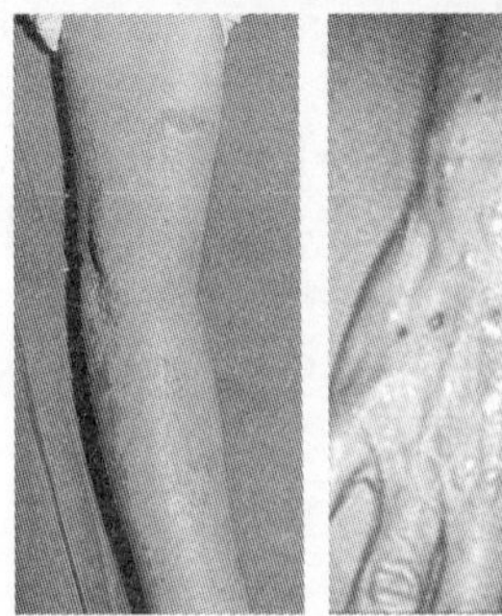

Photo-dermatitis

Erythema, scaling and oedema on the forearm and the back of hands due to an excessive exposure to sunlight on high altitude or along the sea-shore follows *pigmentation, dermatitis, sunburn, redness and inflammation.* Use a sunscreen cream/lotion to protect the skin.

Impetigo

It is of two types: *Bullous Impetigo* and *Impetigo Contagiosa.*

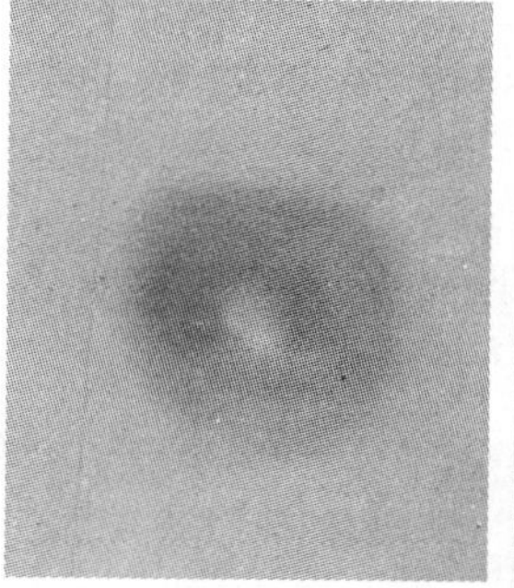

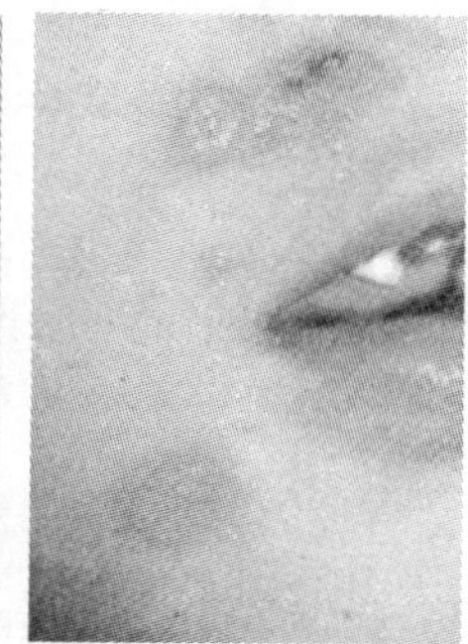

1. A large *bulla* filled with pus due to Pyogenic infection (Pyodermas). It is more common in children on the face, and known as *Bullous Impetigo.*
2. *Impetigo Contagiosa* is a superficial pustule and ulcer with yellowish pusy crust on the face, usually more common in children.

Ecthyma

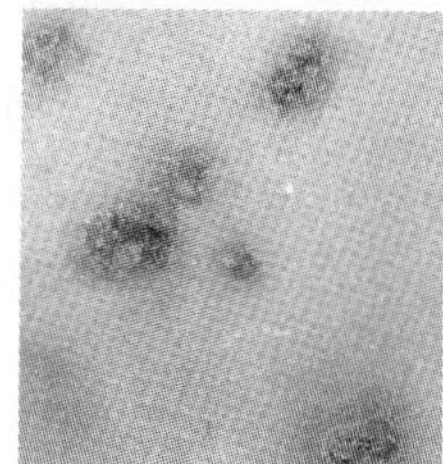

A common disorder among older children or teenagers in which the infection having dark brown or black crusts extend deeper into the dermis. Sometimes, the pus may stain with the blood.

Erysipelas

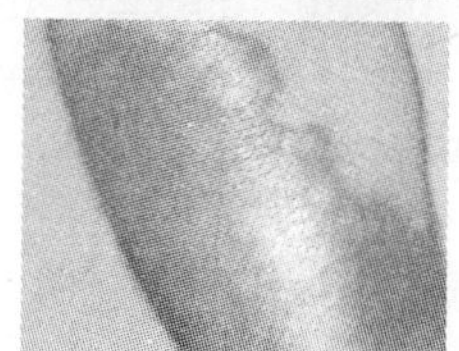

The lesion consists of swelling and redness with raised border, usually warm and tender and sometimes associated with fever.

Acute paronychia

An infection of the nail-fold producing reddish swelling and painful ingrowing of the nail.

Follicitis

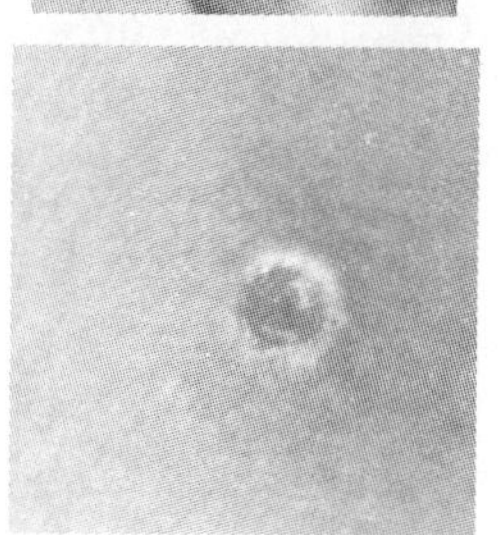

A recurrent infection of the hair follicle with multiple pustular lesions around the hair follicles on the legs, thighs and the beard region of men on the face occurring on the hairy areas of the body.

Eczematoid dermatitis

An infective eczema leading to itching and scaly lesions. The presence of bacteria in lesions may be diagnosed from the pus. Mostly crusting, scaling and papulo-vesicles around the ear or on the nape of the neck discharge pus. Antibiotic treatment (under the advice of a doctor) is recommended. Improved hygiene, avoiding the use of oil, malnutrition and immune deficiency bring relief in this type of infection.

Papulo-nectoric tuberculoid (tuberculosis of the skin)

This disorder of the skin is caused by *mycobacterium* which gets implanted by the blood stream or by a contagious spread. It manifests in various forms:

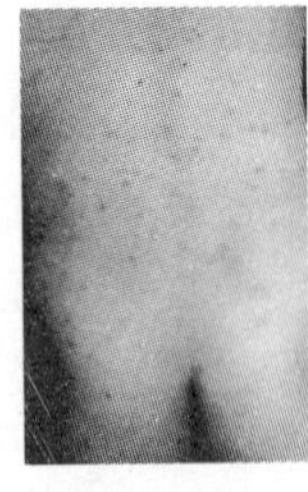

1. **Lupus valgaris:** Group of verrucous plaques involving lesions on the face, buttocks and any other part of the body, leaving a scar.
2. **Tuberculosis verrucose cutis:** Deeply indurated lesions similar to Lupus valgaris, which affects the hands or the feet leaving a scar.
3. **Scrofuloderma:** Multiple sinuses start as an infection of the underlying tissue (such as the lymphnodes, bones and joints) with a thin yellowish pusy discharge.

In case of the **Papulo-necrotic Tuberculoid**, the bacteria spreads in the body producing multiple nodules and papules with necrosis at the centre, especially on the trunk with a scar formation on healing.

Fungal dermatophytosis (nail plate destroyed by fungus)

The nail plate is usually involved by the deposition of fungus under the distal free edge of the nail. In this condition, the nail plate is destroyed by the fungus or white spots appear on the nails. It may become brownish or a discolouration may appear on the thick plate of the nails.

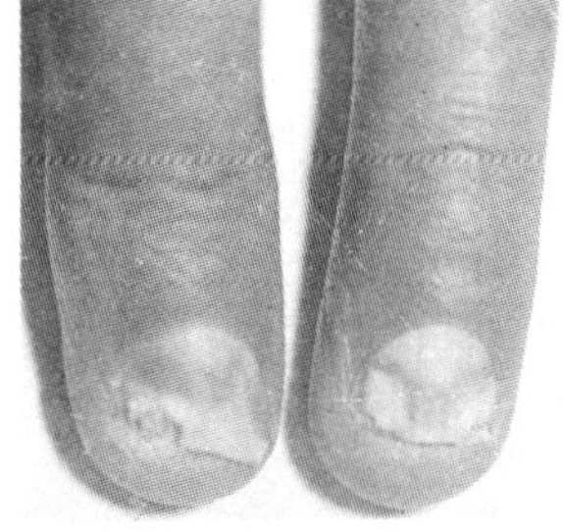

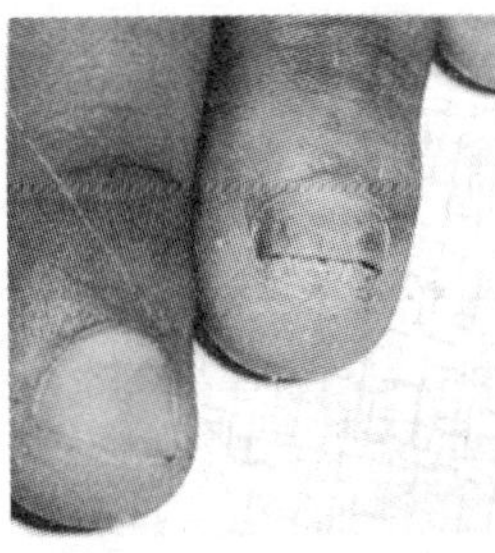

Candidiasis

Candidiasis caused by *Candida albicans* develops in the gastro-intestinal tract. As a result the following disorders are produced:

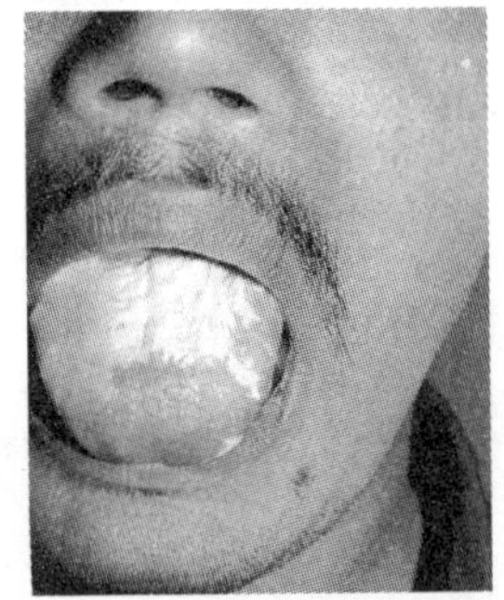

1. *Thrush:* A whitish curd-like deposit on the tongue is common in infants as well as in adults with immune deficiency.
2. *Vulva Vaginitis:* A curd-like whitish deposit on the vagina is produced on the mucosa with redness in the surrounding area or on the glans in the male organ. The vaginal infection can be transmitted to the male partner and vice versa.

Intertriginous candidiasis

Redness and lesions grow in the groin, infra-mammary region in the adult women, between the fingers and at the angles of the mouth among both the sexes of any age group. The trouble is caused by regular soaking of hands in water for a long period which damages the nail fold and the nail plate. When the inflammation is severe, it may ooze pus.

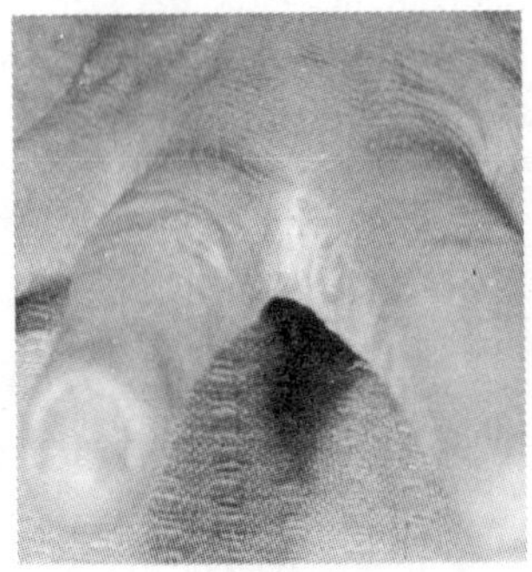

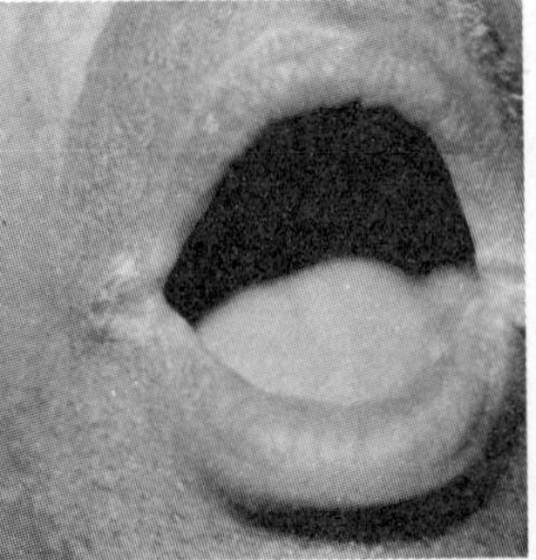

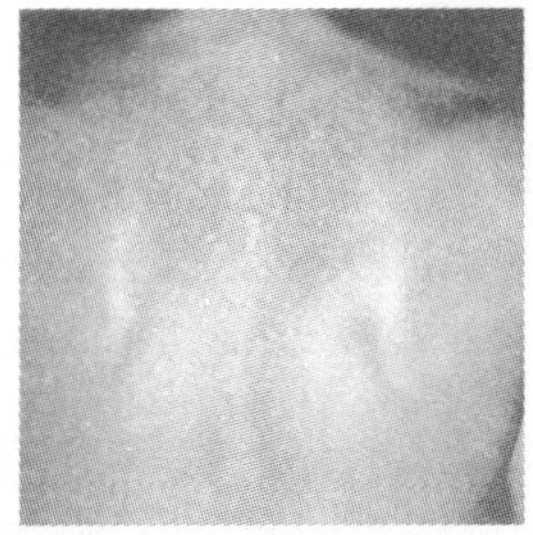

Pityriasis versicolor

A fungal infection which usually starts around the hair follicles on the upper back, shoulders, upper chest and the upper arms. This infection is rare on the neck, face, hands, forearms and the lower limbs of the body. The disease tends to become more extensive in summer.

Molluseum contagiosum

This is caused by a virus, common in children as well as in adults. Skin-coloured, shiny, smooth, infectious lesions 2-10 mm or pinkish papules on the body (sometimes on the shaft of the penis) occur in clusters. The lesions in the genital area are usually caused by sexual contact. The treatment includes cauterisation of the lesions with phenol or trichloroacetic acid in consultation with a doctor.

Scabies

This infectious disease is transmitted from one individual to the other in all ages, usually caused by bite by a wild animal or sometimes of the pet animals such as dog, cat, horse, cattle, etc. Severe itching (more severe at night) lesions are commonly seen on hands, wrists, elbows, axillae, lower part of the abdomen, ankles, thighs, breasts (in females) and the penis and scrotum in the males. The infection sometimes produces *pustule, crusts and lymphadenopathy*. Refer to a doctor for the treatment.

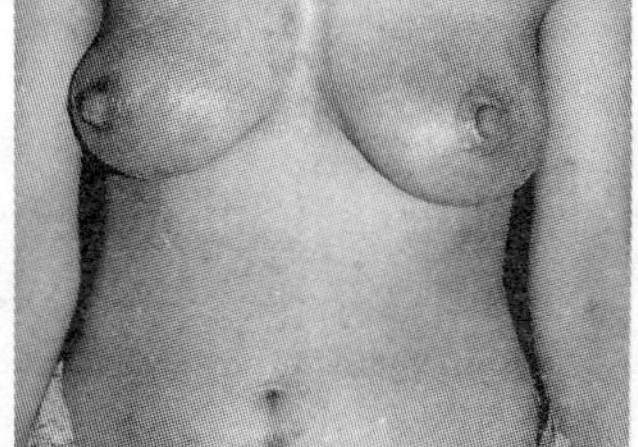

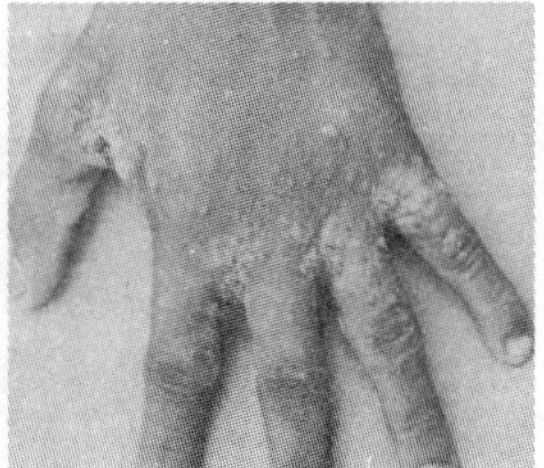

Pediculosis capitis

It is caused by the head louse which infests only the scalp hair. *Pediculosis corporis* is caused by the louse which live in the seams of the clothes and bites the skin. They are usually caused due to poor hygiene. *Pediculosis pubis* infests the hair in the pubic region, axillae, beard, moustache and eyelashes, and many times spreads to the trunk. The nits can be seen sticking to the pubis area. The treatment consists of application of 1% gamma benzene hexachloride or 0.25% malathion. In case of the eyelashes, apply petrolatum to the eyelashes four to five times a day and consult a doctor.

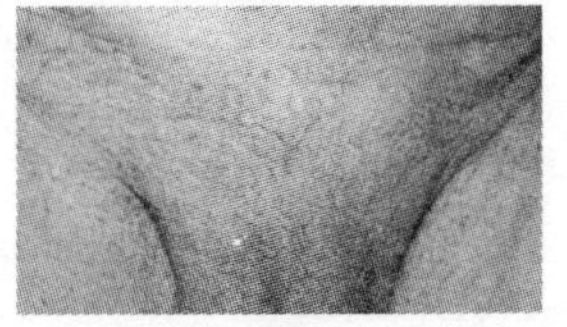

Contact dermatitis

This term is used when the dermatitis is caused by the contact with an agent to which one has developed contact through hypersensitivity. These sensitive agents include shoes, jewellery, particular clothes, cosmetics, a plant or contact with a metal.

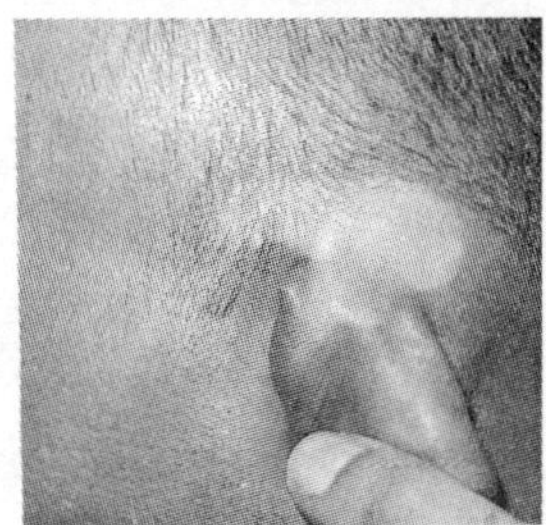

Vitiligo

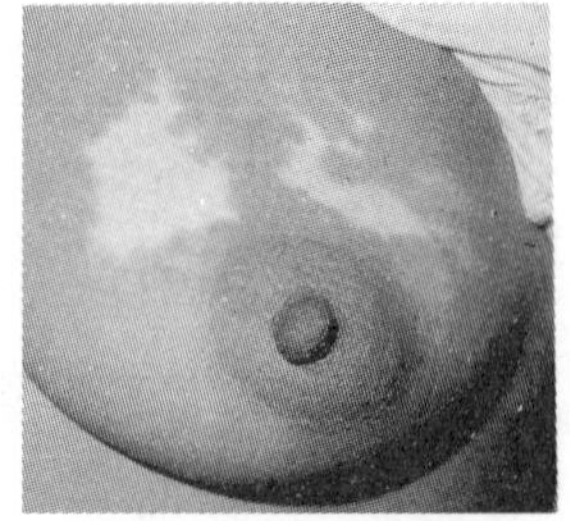

A pigmentary disorder of the skin when the melanocytes in the localised areas of the body stop producing melanin. The lesions vary in shape and size and may appear on any part of the skin on the body and mucous membranes and spread quickly. In most cases, the lesions tend to be localised to the skin of the arms, knees, elbows, ankles and knuckles. Depigmentation on the forehead is caused by the adhesive of the plastic *bindi*, on breasts due to the plastic purse kept under the brassiere, on the fold of the ear by spectacle frames, on the feet by the rubber straps of the slippers and on the waist due to the tight pressure caused by the petticoat string.

Seborrhoeic dermatitis

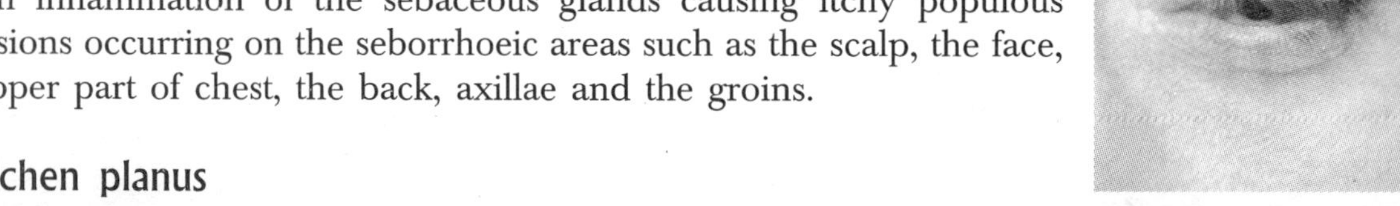

An inflammation of the sebaceous glands causing itchy populous lesions occurring on the seborrhoeic areas such as the scalp, the face, upper part of chest, the back, axillae and the groins.

Lichen planus

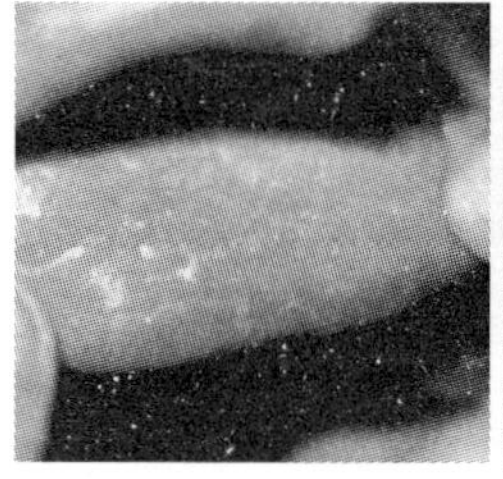

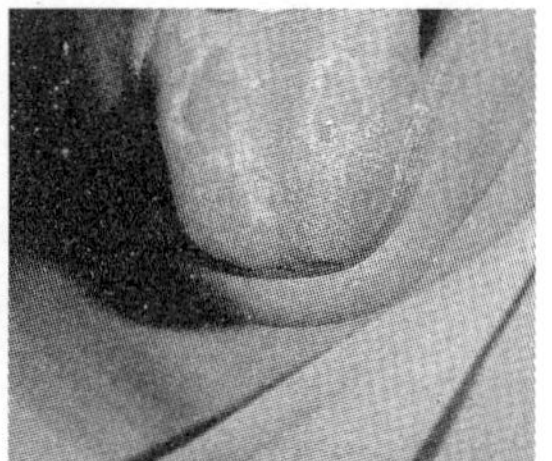

The disease manifests in several forms causing severe itching, violaceous-pink or whitish papules or lesions on the body (forearm, back and legs), on the lower lip, tongue, nail plate, palms and soles and the genitals (on the shaft of the penis and on the glans penis).

Melanocytic naevus

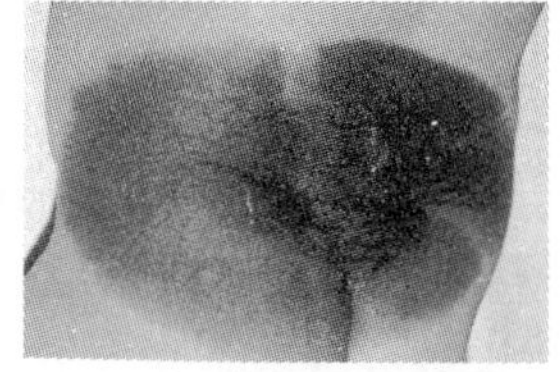

This is also called *pigmentary naevi.* These are small macules or pigmented papules with or without hairs. Cheeks, hands, upper chest, lower back and buttocks are the commonly affected areas. Most naevi can be left untreated. However, a naevus can be excised surgically or with a laser.

Red cheeks

If you have found that your skin reacts to products and shows signs of irritation or redness, you probably have hyper-reactive skin. There are two types of skin that fall into the sensitive skin categories: One that is susceptible to breakouts, and the other that is easily irritated. The irritations come from an overdose of a product or using products that are too harsh. Your skin comes into the category of hyper-sensitive when:

- You are prone to blotchy skin patches.
- Products or cosmetics often cause redness and irritation.
- Skin breaks out with exposure to household cleaners.

- Alpha hydroxy acids and retinols irritate your skin.

Care of a sensitive skin should include getting rid of the triggering factors, using hypoallergenic and fragrance-free cosmetics, etc.

Varicose veins

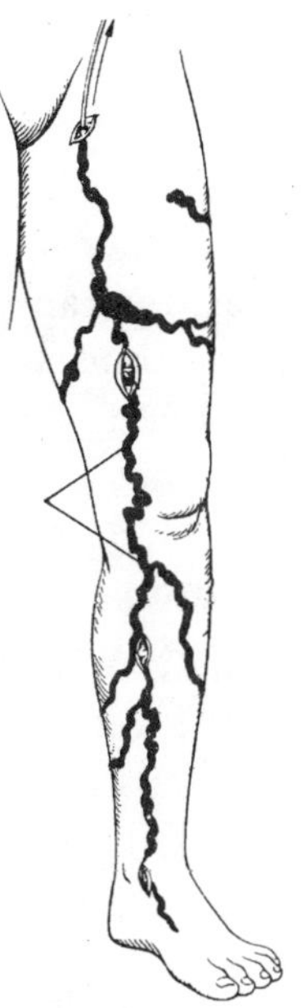

These are caused due to lack of exercise, obesity and standing for long time as a result of which blood circulation in the veins becomes slow causing congestion of the blood. The valves in the veins becomes weak causing discomfort and pain in the legs. People with *varicose veins* first note *swelling* along the course of the veins, followed by *muscle cramps* and a tired feeling in the legs behind the knees. In some cases, skin over the lower part of the leg may break down, forming a large, ugly ulcer, which is often painful especially when *thrombophlebitis* develops in th legs.

One frequent cause of varicose veins is pregnancy, when there is pressure in the pelvis or abdomen and this disease, may slow the flow of blood back to the heart from the lower extremities affecting the weak veins in the genital area. Leg ulcers and varicose veins are also common in older people. Wherever possible, it is wise to have the large twisting veins completely removed by surgery. However, smaller ulcers of the legs may heal without further surgery. Practice of inverted yogic exercises such as *Shirsh asana, Salamba Shirshasana, Sarvangasana* and *Viparitakarani* help the flow of blood towards the heart.

Natural medicines help relieve pain, reduce the size of veins and stop new veins from forming. Here are a few remedies:

- The nutrient strengthens vein walls. A daily dose of 2,000 to 3,000 milligrams of vitamin C is usually recommended (consult doctor for suitable dose).
- A hot and cold bath before bed improves circulation to the legs, preventing varicosities and helping them to heal. Put your feet in the cold water for 30 seconds, then in the very warm water for two minutes. Repeat three times, ending with 30 seconds in cold water.
- Elevate the foot of your bed to relieve pain by improving circulation in your legs during the night. Insert a brick under the foot of the bed.
- Exercise is very useful for people often suffering from varicose veins. Walking or jogging in the water is the best exercise. The pressure of the water on the outside of the legs is effective in pushing the blood out of the legs and into the circulation.
- Avoid wearing high heel shoes.
- Stay away from tight-fitting clothes. Tight garments, particularly a girdle that is too tight or panty that is too constricting in the groin, keep blood pooled in your legs.

- Don't smoke. Smoking may be a risk factor for those with varicose veins.
- Hormonal imbalances (which usually occur with birth control pills) can be a cause of varicose veins.
- Watch your weight. Added body weight means more pressure on your legs. This is the reason pregnant women usually suffer from varicose veins.

Cramps

Calcium is necessary for the nerves and the muscles. When the calcium level in the body drops below a safe level, the nerves become extremely irritable and the muscles go into a spasm. Cramping pains may then be felt in various parts of the body, particularly, in the larger muscles of the legs. But nowhere is calcium more important than in the muscles of the heart. When the calcium level is reduced in the blood stream, the heart loses its power, becomes irregular, and may even stop beating altogether.

Gout

Gout is a type of arthritis, in which throbbing pain often strikes at night, turning the skin red, hot, swollen and tender. High level of uric acid in the blood is a sure sign of gout. If the attack is intensely painful, a powerful (very toxic) drug helps stop the pain by dissolving the uric acid. The following treatments are recommended:

- Drink sufficient amount of water to flush the uric acid crystals out of your system.
- Stop taking alcohol. Alcohol of all types including beer, wine and liquor triggers the body to produce uric acid.
- Taking a tablespoon of apple cider vinegar daily in the morning is very effective to prevent gout attacks.
- Vitamin B_6 helps distribute water in the body to keep all tissues hydrated.
- Apply crushed ice pack if the affected joint is not too tender to touch.
- Avoid high-purine foods, which contribute to higher levels of uric acid.
- Control your high blood pressure, which increases trouble. Consult your doctor for prescribing a medicine to lower your blood pressure, decreasing sodium intake and losing excess weight gradually.

Body and foot odour

You may have a beautiful body, but your whole charm will be lost if your body smells bad. Bad body odour can be an indication of an underlying medical problem and internal cleansing is the best way to correct it. Here are a few suggestions and precautions for detoxifying your body and getting rid of body odour. The main cause of body odour is a combination of perspiration and bacteria. Scrubbing your body with soap or a body wash and water will wash both culprits away. The best type of wash for the body is a deodorant soap to fight bacteria.

- Drinking lots of water everyday helps the body dilute and get rid of odour-causing toxins. You may add a squeeze of lemon juice to each glass, which helps the body detoxify.
- The herb goldenseal can kill the toxic bacteria in the intestines and can help reduce the body odour. Follow the dosage recommended on the label. Probiotics (a food supplement) help maintain the health of the intestines and reduce the bad intestinal bacteria that can trigger a strong body odour.
- Massage your body. Brushing the skin with a natural-bristle dry skin brush stimulates the skin, improves circulation, removes old dead skin cells and can help the body get rid of odour causing toxins. Start brushing with short, brisk strokes with the front and back of your arms, moving from the fingertips towards the armpits and always towards the heart. Then brush the front and back of your legs starting at your feet (including bottom) and brushing upward. Finally move up brushing gently the inner thighs, the pelvic area, buttocks, abdomen, lower back, chest and upper back without letting the brush get wet. Brushing should never be painful.
- Keep calm. Getting sexually excited or feeling anxious and nervous will make you perspire more. Meditation and practicing deep breathing should be your daily routine.
- Watch what you eat. Extracts of proteins and oils from certain foods and spices remain in your body's excretions and secretions for hours and can impart an odour. Avoid eating fish, cumin, curry and garlic.

Foot Odour: One of the best ways to get rid of bad smell from the feet is to get rid of bacteria. If you have tried various home remedies for foot odour and your feet still smell, see a podiatrist, have a physical examination and see a naturopathic physician to undergo a detoxification program which will help rid the body of toxic substances that can contribute to foot odour. Here are some home recipes to relieve foot odour:

- Put ¼–1 cup of vinegar (according to the condition) in a basin of water and add to it a few drops of strong anti-bacterial liquid grapefruit seed extract. Soak your feet for 15-20 minutes a day for one to two weeks until the bacteria are dead and the odour vanishes. Do not soak your feet in the liquid if you have areas of broken skin on your feet.
- Herbs play an important role to relieve foot odour. Natural anti-perspirant herbs, sage or coriander stop foot odour. Apply it to the soles of your feet once or twice a day. Baking soda is another natural anti-perspirant that can help prevent foot odour.
- Soak feet in a basin of water added to which are a few drops of thyme essential oil, which reduce unpleasant smells.
- Stay cool. Sweat glands in your feet, similar to those in your armpits and palms respond to emotions. Stress, whether good or bad triggers excessive sweating and in turn increases bacterial activity in your shoes leading to extra odour.
- Watch what you eat. Avoid eating spicy or pungent smelling foods such as onions, peppers, garlic or scallions.

Burns, blisters and scarring

You can treat most first-degree burns, like most sunburns and scalds, which are red and painful. The second-degree burns include severe sunburns or burns caused by brief contact with oven coils; they blister, ooze and are painful. Third-degree burns are charred and white or creamy coloured, and are caused by chemical reaction, electricity current or prolonged contact with hot surfaces. They require immediate medical help. Other burns that demand doctor's help include burns to the face, hands, feet, pelvic, pubic areas, eyes, burns showing signs of infection (blister filled with greenish or brownish fluid), a burn that becomes hot and turns red and any burn that doesn't heal in ten days to two weeks. Signs of infection such as increased redness, pain, swelling, pus and spreading red streaks usually start appearing two-three days after the burn. Electrical or chemical burns should always be treated by a doctor because they may be worse than they appear. Following natural measures to treat the burn are recommended:

- Good diet and supplement of vitamin E, vitamin C, zinc and beta-carotene help speed recovery and promote wound healing.
- Leaf of aloe (herbal plant) is the best remedy for minor kitchen burns. Cut off a leaf of the plant, pull off its outer skin and apply paste directly on the burn.
- Gently wrap the burn in a clean, dry cloth to avoid infection.
- Starting 24 hours after you burn, wash your injury gently with soap and water or a mild betadine solution once a day (better have consultation with your doctor).
- In case of blisters that pop, clean the area with soap and water, then smooth on a little antibiotic ointment.
- Essential oil of lavender witnesses amazing healing of burns. Mix witch-hazel and clean water in equal quantity and add to it a few drops of essential oil of lavender. Store the bottle in a cool, dark place and spray it on after shaking thoroughly.

Blisters: It is a small area of broken cells where leaking fluid has pooled and separated the outer layer of the skin from the underlying tissue. The essential oil of lavender regenerates the skin cells. Lavender is one of the few essential oils that you can apply directly to the skin without diluting it in carrier oil. Just put a few drops of pure oil (not a fragrance or perfume) on the blister. Then cover it with an adhesive bandage. Apply oil two to three times a day until the blister is healed. A blister is infected when the fluid oozing from it is not clear like water or when it has some odour to it. People who very often suffer from blisters on the back of their heels should wear socks, and shoes without heels. Always sprinkle powder before wearing socks.

Scarring: Scars are usually not a threat to physical health, but if you have a scar that appears unattractive, you must consult a dermatologist or a plastic surgeon. Keloids are hard, firm masses of scar tissue that grow above the skin surface and may be painful or itchy. If you develop a keloid, see a dermatologist about treatments for removal. Putting a few drops of undiluted essential oil of lavender on the skin immediately after an injury or a surgery can prevent excessive scarring.

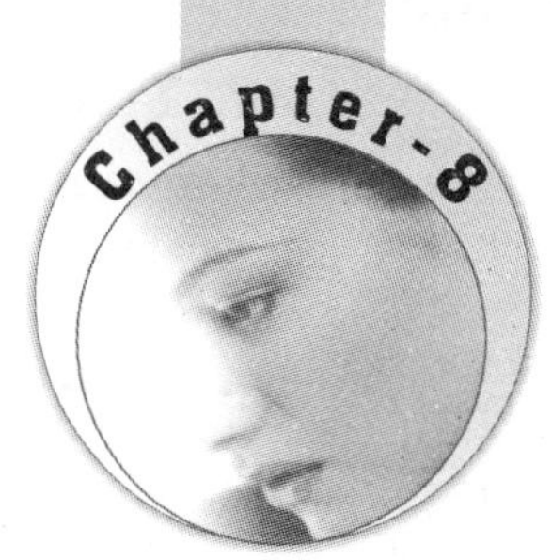

Therapies for Skin Beauty

Some of the therapies are described below:

Ozone Therapy

It includes producing alkaline rays used for both scalp and facial skin treatments (such as itchy scalp, dandruff, acne, pimples and busting pusy infection). This therapy is performed by using anti-allergic, antiseptic and sterilised powder.

Micro Therapy

This is a power massing therapy to treat ageing skin showing signs of laughing lines, frown lines, crow's feet. This therapy helps to improve the blood circulation, stimulate nerves and muscles, regenerate cells and tissues, face lifting and promotes the elastin fibres of the skin.

High Frequency Therapy

In primary action of this treatment, thermal heat is produced due to rapid vibration but without muscular contractions. The beneficial result of this therapy includes relieving dark circles and puffiness under the eyes, and rejuvenates crow's feet and shrunken eyes.

Derma Brasion

Various skin problems are solved by this therapy in which layers of the skin damaged due to acne, scars, blemishes and pigmentation marks causing an uneven tone are removed. The various benefits include levelling the surface of the skin, reducing the scars and removing tanning.

Corrective line massage treatment

It is basically meant for mature and oily skin. With age, fine lines develop on the skin, which result in loosening of the skin, puffiness, etc. To give firmness or tightness to the skin, corrective line massage or treatments are done in men and women above 30 years of age. This can be done in two processes:

- **Mild Process:** This is given by hands in case of light lines on the skin.
- **Strong Process:** This is given with the help of toning and lifting gadgets in case of sharp lines.

Uneven-tone treatment

Uneven-tone skin is caused due to improper blood circulation, effect of UVA rays (cool) and UVB rays (hot). Mostly uneven-tone skin is found in T-Zone and C-Zone of the facial skin.

Procedure: The following procedure should be applied for the treatment:

- Apply rose water on the skin.
- Give alkaline wash to the skin.
- Apply softening milk. Remove whiteheads by the process of suction and blackheads from all over the face.
- Apply oligo ampoule all over the face, followed by the application of oligo mask on it.
- Remove face pack by gentle massage. Prepare paste by mixing Derma Peel and Papaya enzymes and Bio Peel Acid in hot water. Apply the paste on the affected area, followed by brushing clockwise and anti-clockwise to clear the skin. Do not spread the paste all over the face.
- After cleansing the skin use cold spray all over the face.
- Use Derma brazing gadget for strong procedure.

Pigmentation treatment

Pigmentation on the skin is caused due to:

- Loss of water.
- Improper blood circulation.
- Mental tension.
- Lack of sleep or disturbed sleep.

Procedure:

- Alkaline wash with steam.
- Softening milk and suction.
- Application of Biorrubin Ampoule and oligo mask.
- Application of derma peeling on chin, upper lip and nose. Do not use brushing on these areas.
- Apply lymphatic cream according to the skin.
- Gently massage and apply Alpha Hydroxy Acid pack.

Custom-designed face masks

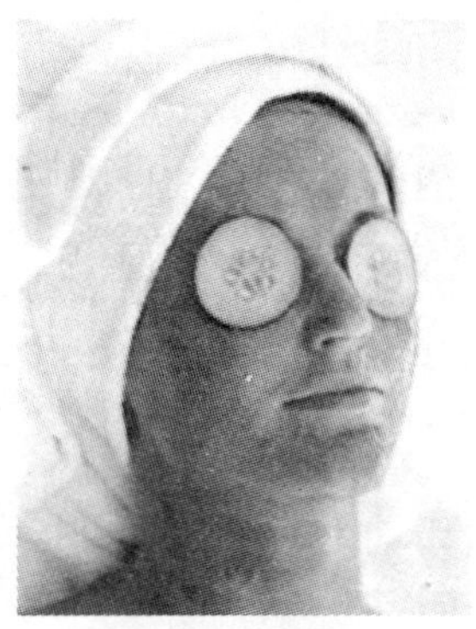

These face masks are usually prepared from fresh fruits, vegetables, milk, yoghurt or eggs. They are left on the face for 10–15 minutes. Fresh fruits can be crushed or sliced and applied to the face for a mild astringent, stimulating mask. Crushed banana mask is useful for dry and sensitive skin, leaving it soft and smooth. Strawbery mask is a highly effective astringent.

Vegetables too are mild astringents and have excellent soothing qualities. The most beneficial vegetables are tomatoes and cucumbers. Carrot juice, rich in vitamin A is used for nourishing the skin. Basil *(tulsi)* leaves are a potent skin tonic. Coriander *(dhania)* is a carminative and a cooling agent. Garlic *(lahsan)* has an antiseptic, drawing property which helps cure several skin diseases. Lemon, rich in vitamin C, has acidic properties and is used in bleaching and astringent lotions. Onion juice prevents blemishes when applied on the skin mixed with honey. Potato has cleansing and drawing properties. It clears the skin and removes the puffiness of the eyes.

White of the egg can be beaten until fluffy and applied to the face as a mask. It has a tightening effect and clears the skin. Yoghurt and buttermilk are used for masks on all types of skin. Yoghurt contains certain valuable enzymes and is used as a base for cleansing and face masks. Buttermilk has a mild astringent, cleansing action which leaves the skin feeling refreshed. Honey is used for toning, which leaves a tightening and hydrating effect on the skin. Vitamin A is useful for dry skin and cures acne. Vitamin B promotes the health of the skin. Vitamin C heals acne and pimples. Vitamin D has a healing effect on the skin. Vitamin E is said to have healing properties and Vitamin F counteracts dry and chapped skin.

Marigold and Rose flowers are a rich source of beauty. Marigold cures varicose veins and various circulatory troubles. As a lotion, a marigold infusion (petals only) is very useful for an oily skin and complexion and helps cure eczema and ringworms. Rose petals are a rich source of Vitamin E. Rose water is widely used in skin tonics and creams. Oils play an important role in beauty care. The range of oils is so vast to cover the entire top-to-toe beauty. Almond, coconut, sesame, castor, clove and cinnamon are commonly used varieties of oils to enhance skin and hair beauty. Almond oil is used for face massage because it improves complexion, prevents wrinkles around the eyes and removes eye make-up. Coconut oil, when mixed with camphor cures skin diseases and makes the hair healthy. Sesame oil softens rough skin and enhances the growth of hair. Olive oil (when massaged) nourishes the skin and makes the hair healthy and glossy.

Skin cleansing, moisturising and toning

Almost every skin care product will fall into one of the three main categories. It will cleanse, tone or nourish. Some preparations will fit into more than one category, which cleanse and tone or cleanse and nourish. Moisturisers normally come into the nourishing category.

Cleansing creams

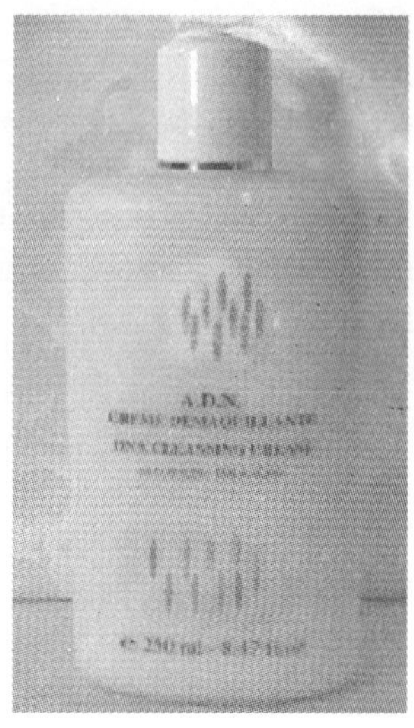

These are the first and amongst the most important of the skin care products. Soap is a cleanser although not recommended when it comes to cleanse skin especially when make-up has been used. If you must use soap, choose a mild one, baby soap or a type specially designed for the face. A washing gel is recommended for washing the face. But in addition to soap and water, you will still need to use a cosmetic cleanser. Cosmetic cleansers are available in many forms: ordinary cold cream, liquefying cream, cleansing milk and lotion. All cleansers dissolve make-up and remove dirt, dust and grime from the pores. Some are slightly astringent or refreshing and these are usually intended for quick daytime cleansing before reapplying fresh make-up. The creams and emulsions are more commonly used at night when it is very essential to deep-cleanse the skin to remove every trace of make-up (including stale make-up) and grime. Generally, rich creams are best for dry skins and liquefying creams or cleansing lotions are the best for the oily type of skins. There are special cleansers for blemished skins, which tend to have a drying effect.

Cucumber juice cleansing cream

Collect ingredients, such as: 3 teaspoons (tsp.) bees-wax, 4 tsp. coconut oil, 5 tsp. olive oil, 4 tsp. cucumber juice, 1 tsp. glycerine, a pinch of borax powder and a drop of green colouring. Mix oils and wax into an enamel bowl and melt slowly over a pan of boiling water to save the useful contents from burning. Simultaneously, heat the cucumber juice, glycerine, colouring and borax in a separate bowl. Ensure that the borax dissolves thoroughly. When the contents of both the bowls are melted and are warm, add water drop by drop to the oil, stirring continuously. Now remove it from heat and beat until the mixture thickens and cools. Keep the cream in the refrigerator as cucumber juice spoils quickly. Always make the cream in small quantity.

Rose water cleansing lotion

Collect ingredients, such as: 1 tbsp. bees-wax or white paraffin wax, 1 tbsp. emulsifying wax, 4 tbsp. mineral oil, 6 tbsp. rose water, ½ tbsp. borax powder and a few drops of rose oil (perfume). Melt the waxes and oil together, and at the same time, heat the water and borax and make sure that the borax is completely dissolved. Remove both the bowls from heat and pour water into the oil. Continue stirring until a white cream begins to form. Add a few drops of rose oil when the mixture begins to cool. Carry on beating until the mixture thickens.

Moisturising creams

Most moisturising creams and lotions have low oil but high moisture content, which supply moisture and oil to the skin. They protect the skin by combating the drying effects of cold weather, sun, hair dryer, central heating, radiant fires, dust, fog and tinted cosmetics. Apply moisturiser after cleansing and toning and always before a make-up. If you are not wearing a make-up, a thin film of moisturiser is helpful under the face pack for a dry skin. It can be used in place of a skin food on a young skin or a youthful normal or oily skin, which needs some nourishment.

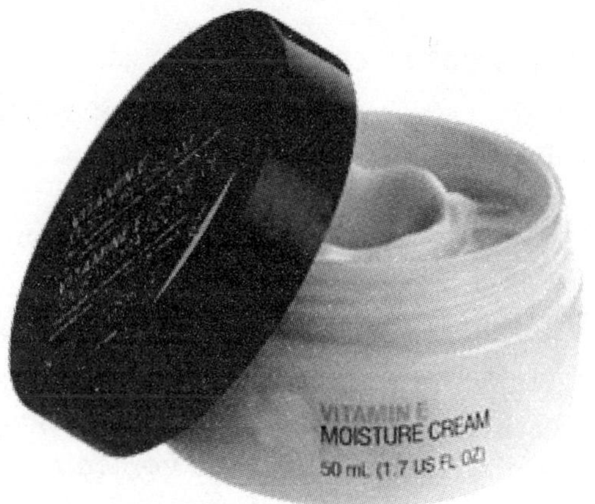

Almond Oil Moisturising Cream

Collect ingredients, such as: 2 tsp. bees-wax, 1 tsp. emulsifying wax, 5 tsp. almond oil and a few drops of lavender oil. Melt over hot water, both the bees-wax and emulsifying wax in a bowl. When melted, mix the almond oil to it. In another bowl, heat water at the same temperature and slowly add to the melted waxes and oils, stirring all the time. Remove the mixture from the heat and continue stirring. When cool, add the lavender oil.

Honey Moisturising Cream

Collect ingredients, such as: 3 tbsp. lanolin, ½ tsp. honey, 1 tsp. lecithin, 4 tbsp. warm water and a few drops of perfume. Heat lanolin, honey and lecithin in a bowl. Now mix to it some warm water, stirring constantly. This is one of the creams which need not be refrigerated.

Nourishing creams

These include all skin foods whether they are oil-based or of the moisturising types and whether they are light and immediately absorbed or heavy and sticky needing to be massaged into the skin. Hormone creams and lotions, vitamin products, serum ampoules, anti-wrinkle creams and lotions, biologically-active preparations containing placental extracts and other laboratory-prepared ingredients all come into the nourishing group. What your skin needs depends on its type and the age. The more dry and mature it is, the more active product is required. An ordinary skin food will supply all that the skin needs in the way of oils and lubricating ingredients throughout the twenties and thirties and possibly until menopause.

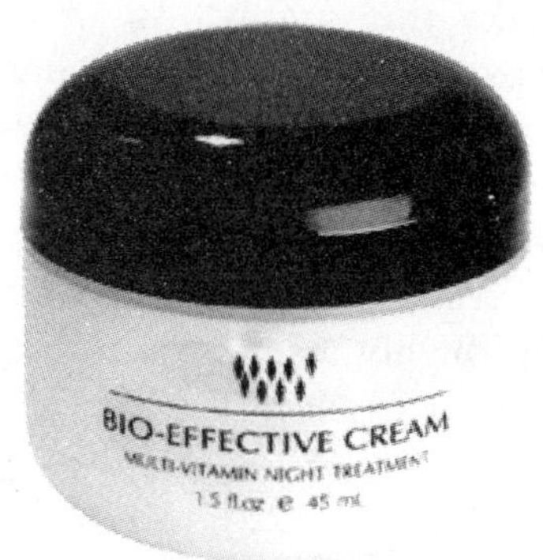

During menopause and afterwards, when the body's supply of hormones and other vital elements slow down then creams and lotions containing hormones, special extracts, serums, rich creams containing vitamins and concentrated oils may all help to give the skin a more youthful appearance. Given below are a few cleansing, moisturising and toning home-preparations you can try yourself.

Cocoa butter cream

Collect ingredients, such as: 2 tbsp. cocoa butter, 2 tbsp. emulsifying wax, 1 tbsp. bees-wax, 4 tbsp. sesame oil and 1 tbsp. almond oil. When all the ingredients are completely melted, remove from the heat and stir until the cream is cool, adding a few drops of perfume. The cream leaves the skin smooth without being greasy.

Vitamin cream

Collect ingredients, such as: 1 tbsp. bees-wax, 1 tbsp. emulsifying wax, 1 tbsp. lanolin and 2 capsules of vitamin E. Melt waxes and lanolin on slow heat, stirring constantly. Add to it vitamin E capsules till the contents of the capsules are mixed thoroughly.

Vegetable cream

Collect ingredients, such as: 2 tbsp. bees of wax, 4 tbsp. emulsifying wax, 3 tsp. lanolin, 4 tbsp. almond oil, 4 tbsp. sesame oil, 2 tbsp. avocado oil, 2 tbsp. safflower oil, 2 tbsp. sunflower, 5 tbsp. water, ½ tsp. borax powder and a few drops of amber oil. Mix and melt the waxes and oils together over a water bath. In a separate bowl, dissolve the borax in warm water. Now add water to the oils and beat until the cream cools. It leaves no sign of grease when applied but gives the skin a satiny sheen.

Rose water

This was discovered by an Arabian in the tenth century. It is easy to make on your own. Mix two tablespoons of the essence of roses in four litres of purified water and shake thoroughly. To make the gypsy rose water, put two handfuls of dark rose petals into a jar containing one litre of water and 200 gms of sugar. Keep the mixture for 24 hours, shake thoroughly, then strain and store in a cool place.

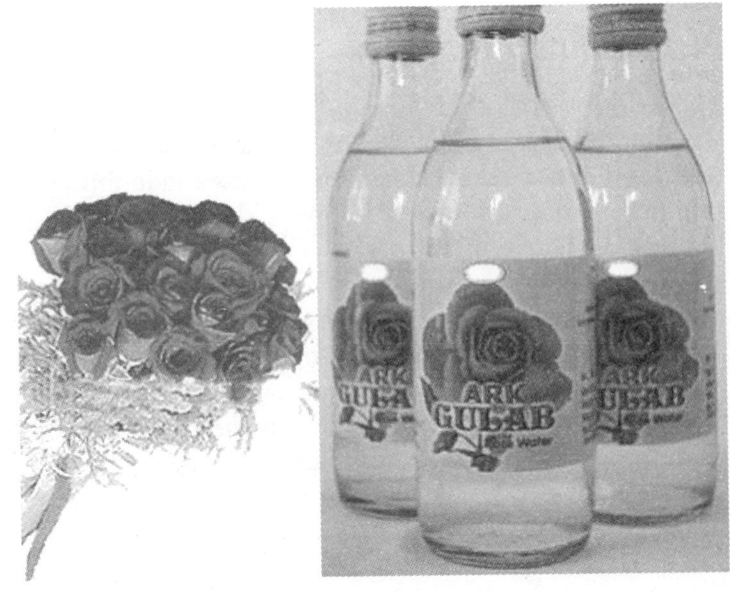

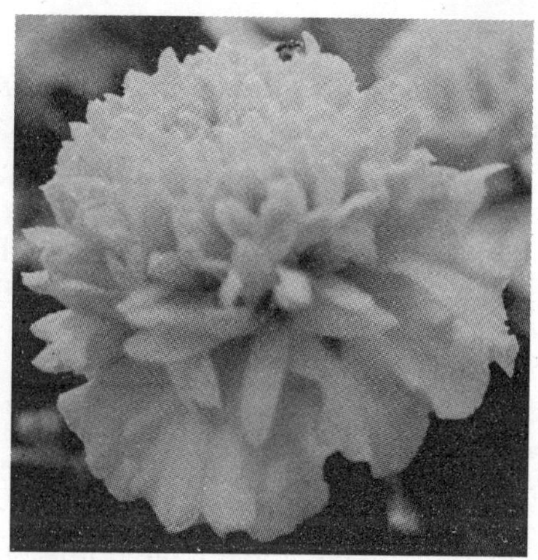

Marigold skin tonic

Mix two dried or three fresh marigold flowers to ½ litre water. Leave for 10 to 12 hours. Mix to it two tablespoons of witch-hazel. It is useful for greasy and spotty skin.

Vinegar skin tonic

Collect ingredients, such as: ½ cup cider vinegar (or wine), ½ tsp. cloves, 1 tbsp. lavender, 1 tbsp. rose petals, 1 tbsp. rosemary and 2 tbsp. rose or orange flower water. The skin has an acid mantle and vinegar being acidic restores it. Always use diluted vinegar in the ratio one part to eight parts of water.

Toning

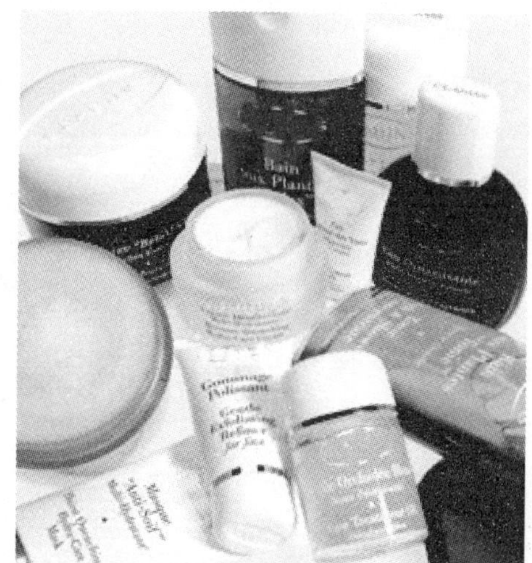

Toners are intended to close pores, freshen the complexion and refine the skin. These are used after cleansing and before a make-up to ensure a smooth matt finish, and also after cleansing and before applying skin food at night. Toning products include skin freshener, skin tonic, astringent lotion, milk, flower extract, herbal and camphor lotions, witch-hazel and rose water. If you have a dry skin, you should use a mild toning lotion such a skin freshener or a flower water (preferably rose water). Any type of skin tonic or skin freshener can be used on normal skins, whereas an astringent lotion or milk or camphor lotion benefit when used on oily skins. An astringent will close up pores and prevent oiliness seeping through make-up. Do not choose a lotion which is too astringent, this may stimulate the sebaceous glands into producing yet more oil.

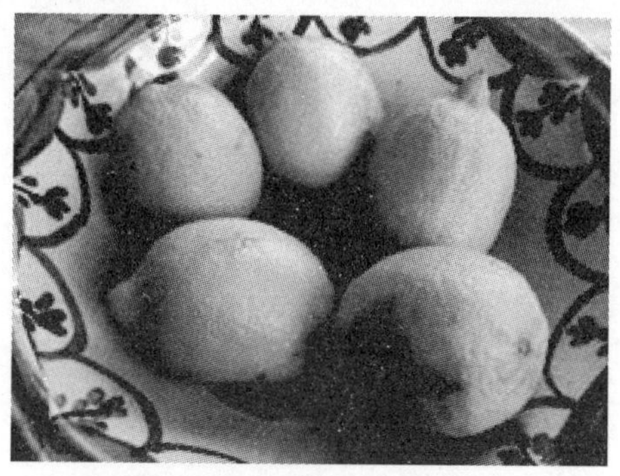

Lemon astringent

Collect ingredients, such as: 4 tbsp. lemon juice, ½ tsp peppermint extract, 8 tbsp. witch-hazel and 2 tbsp. alcohol. Mix all the ingredients together in a large bottle and store for 24 hours, strain and use.

Honey astringent

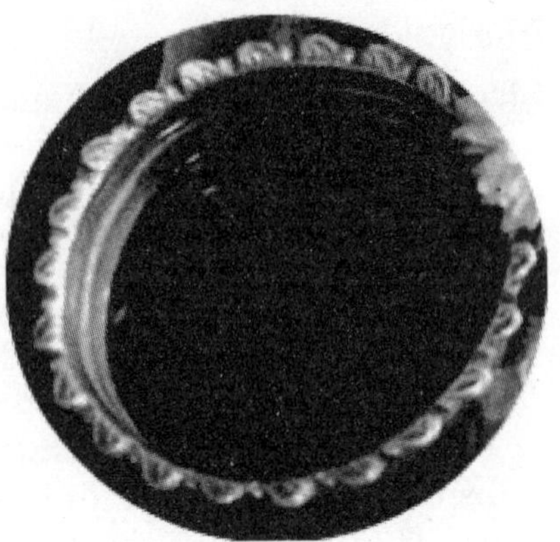

Collect ingredients, such as: 8 tbsp. sandalwood oil, 1 tsp. bergamot oil *(zabir ka tel)*, 1/4 tsp. lavender oil, 1/8 tsp. clove oil, 4 tbsp. rose water, 4 tbsp. orange flower water, 1 tbsp. honey and a pinch of musk or sandalwood chips. Mix all the ingredients together in an airtight jar and keep for two weeks, shake it daily. Bergamot oil helps in tanning the skin.

Camphor astringent

Collect ingredients, such as: 1/2 cup each of rose water, witch-hazel and distilled water. Add to it 1 tbsp. camphor spirit, 2 drops blue colouring and a pinch of alum. Shake it in a large bottle, strain and use to tighten and tone the skin. This lotion can also be used as an aftershave lotion by men.

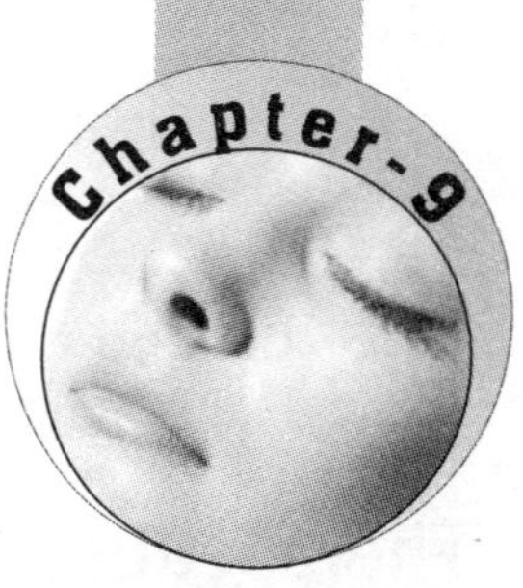

Detox : The Best Way to Get a Radiant Skin

The present century lifestyle places high demands to look after your body. To eliminate toxins, a regular deep cleansing of the skin and hair is essential. You need a beauty detox if:

- You are getting breakouts on the face or on the back of the body.
- The skin on the face and the body is very dry and looks chalky.
- You have dark shadows or circles or puffiness around the eyes.
- The skin looks bumpy on upper arms.
- Skin looks grey and lifeless.
- Hair is dry, brittle and dull.
- Your body feels no energy and you have a poor blood circulation and suffer from cold hands and feet.
- You have cellulite.

Easy ways to give your body a beauty detox

1. **Massage:** It leaves a miraculous effect for improving the blood circulation and lymph drainage to banish cellulite.
2. **Aroma treatment:** This is done mixing up your own blend with 10 ml of a carrier oil such as sweet almond oil and not more than five drops of a pure essential oil such as lemon, juniper or grapefruit to massage as long as it takes the oil to be absorbed on the areas of the body such as your hips, butt, thigh and abdomen, once a day.
3. **Spa type massage:** This helps in good blood circulation if applied after a bath while the skin is still damp and warm. Seal in the oil by smoothing on a body contouring cream.
4. **Body brushing:** This is good for busting cellulite, which smoothes and firms the skin. Do not neglect your back. Brush up your back, legs and arms towards your heart in a circular, clockwise movement through your tummy, preferably in the morning before taking a bath.
5. **Face masking:** It is a good flush out and helps to clear a congested skin using stimulating ingredients such as rosemary, eucalyptus and herbs, leaving a rehydrating effect on dry as well as oily skin. Mask your skin for 5–20 minutes depending upon the condition. The perfect time to mask your face is before retiring to bed at night.

6. **Repairing your hair:** Masks put the shine back into dull hair. Detox shampoos are readily available in the market, which deep cleanse the hair and reduce damage from free radicals.
7. **Bathing eases tension:** Epsom salt bath helps your skin to eliminate toxins. Fill the bath tub up to your neck and roll in it for 20 minutes, breathing deeply.

Therapeutic value of baths

To stimulate the vitality of the body and increase your skin beauty, use water in various ways, at varying temperatures in the form of a pack or a bath. The application of cold water to the abdomen—the seat of most diseases helps to lower the body heat and stimulate the nervous system.

Hydrotherapy offers a simple natural method of abating several body disorders without harmful side-effects. A hip bath and application of wet packs leaves a relaxing effect, revives the dead skin and helps to maintain the physical beauty of the body as well as keeps you healthy. Remember, a healthy body is always beautiful. The application of cold packs to the surface of the body draws the blood from the congested interior to the skin, relaxes its minute blood vessels and opens the skin pores. It facilitates the escape of heat from the body and keeps the body temperature below the danger point by promoting heat radiation through the skin.

A patient suffering from a skin disorder should be familiar with the temperature of the water used. The temperature of water ranging between 4.5–15.5°C is said to be cold, between 15.5–21°C as cool, between 21–32°C as tepid, the temperature between 32–38°C as warm and between 38–43°C is considered hot. Above 43°C temperature, the water loses its therapeutic value and is destructive for the skin. *Hydrotherapy is much more preferable than antipyretics,* which lower the resistance of the body. *Antipyretics* lower the body metabolism and resistance, while *hydrotherapy* increases the body metabolism.

Wet packs

Wet packs may be applied to any part of the body. The different types of wet packs include *Full sheet Pack, Spanish Mantle, Body Pack, Abdominal Pack, Chest Pack, Scotch Pack, Throat Pack, T. Pack, Leg Pack, Foot Pack and Hip Pack.* Wet packs help to lower the high temperature, raise a subnormal temperature, relieve the inner congestions, promote elimination, relieve pain and stimulate the sluggish blood circulation of the body.

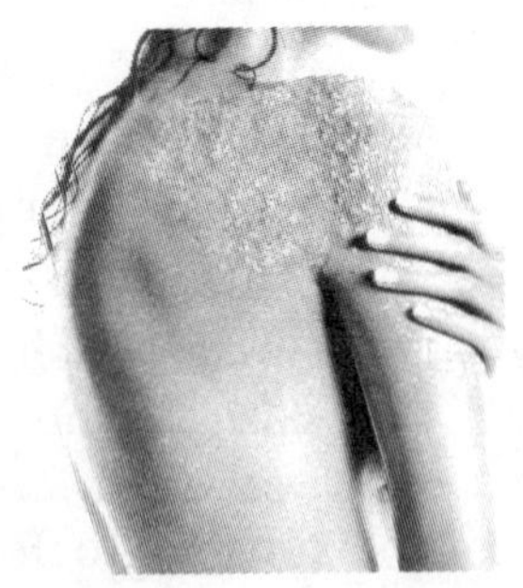

Mud and clay packs

Mud and clay was used extensively for remedial purposes in the ancient times, and with the people going back to Nature, it is again in the spotlight. The best way to apply clay packs is to take **yellow** or still better the **Blue Potter's Clay.** Mix it in warm water until it is reduced to a smooth paste and apply it, until it dries. Mud and clay packs have beneficial results because the cool moisture in and under the pack relaxes the pores of the skin, draws the blood to the surface, relieves inner congestions and pain and promotes heat radiations and elimination of morbid matter.

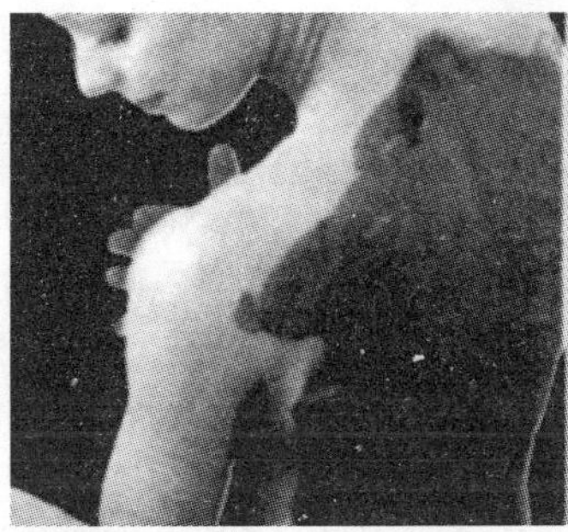

Hip bath

A hip bath is one of the most useful forms of hydrotherapy. As the name suggests, this mode of treatment involves only the hips and the abdominal region below the navel, in a special type of tub filled with water in such a way that it covers the hips and reaches upto the navel when the patient sits in it. *A hip bath is given in cold, hot, neutral and alternate temperatures.*

1. **Cold hip bath:** The water temperature should vary between 10–18°C and the duration of this bath is about 30 minutes. Rub the abdomen briskly from the navel downwards and across the body, with a coarse wet cloth. Undertake moderate exercises after the hip bath to warm the body, which improves the digestive system and helps to reduce the extra flesh from the hips and the abdomen. A cold hip bath is a routine treatment in most disorders and relieves constipation, indigestion, obesity, helps the eliminative organs to function properly, cures uterine problems like irregular menstruation, uterine infection, pelvic inflammation, piles, hepatic congestion, chronic congestion of prostate glands, seminal weakness, impotency, sterility, ovarian displacement, dilation of the stomach and colon, diarrhoea, dysentery, haemorrhage of the bladder and many other problems which affect the beauty and personality of a human.
2. **Neutral bath:** This is a bath in which the temperature of the water varies between 32–36°C. Avoid friction to the abdomen in this case. This hip bath helps to relieve all acute and sub-acute inflammatory conditions.
3. **Hot hip bath:** This bath is generally taken for eight to ten minutes at a water temperature of 40–45°C. Do not apply friction to the abdomen in this bath. Place a cold compress on the head while taking the bath. A cold shower bath is taken immediately after the hot bath for better results.
4. **Hot and cold hip bath:** This is also known as *revulsive hip bath.* The patient should sit in the hot tub for five minutes, then in the cold tub for three minutes or for 10–20 minutes. The temperature of water in the hot tub should vary between 40–45°C and in cold water tub between 10–18°C. The treatment should end with sprinkling of cold water on the hips. This bath relieves chronic inflammatory conditions of the pelvic region such as ovaritis, salpingitis and cellulitis.
5. **Epsom salt bath:** Fill the bath tub with about 135 litres of hot water at 40°C in which 1 to 1.5 kg of epsom salt should be dissolved. Lie down in the tub immersing the trunk, thighs and legs for 15–20 minutes. The best time to take this bath is just before

retiring to bed. This bath is very useful for skin beauty and disorders of the kidney and bladder.

6. **Steam bath:** This is also known as *Sauna Bath.* It is one of the most important water treatments which induces perspiration. *Sauna helps lose a couple of kilogrammes, but you may put them again if you eat or drink immediately after the bath.* Do not drink anything for atleast one hour after taking this bath. Sauna, alongwith yogic exercise and a good diet, can do wonders in reducing the body weight. Sauna is a place to relax and to lie down alone and speechless—in short, to exercise 15 minutes in a Sauna is equivalent to running two kilometres. Toxins are eliminated through the skin by a Sauna bath which helps cure many skin problems like acne, dull, lifeless complexion, etc. Sauna bath is also recommended in clearing cellulitis. The dress worn at the time of Sauna session is generally briefs and bras or swim suit. A bare body will reap more benefit than a covered one. Women generally feel shy, but gradually, they overcome their shyness because persons taking a steam bath are only interested in their own bodies. Heat penetrates more if you sit in the steam chamber. Saunas are not conducive to hair, so better wrap the hair in a towel when having this kind of a bath.
7. **Sea water bath:** It helps to cleanse the skin, firm the muscles, stimulate the circulation and tone up the system. Sea water dries the skin and the hair. After taking bath in sea water, wash yourself with fresh water and rub a little almond oil on the skin.
8. **Tap water bath:** This is good for the skin depending upon the skin type and the hardness or softness of water. If your skin is extremely dry, washing face in hard water will not be helpful. The salt and calcium in water will leave the skin dry. Use a water softener such as a bath salt or oil which will help to counteract this effect. Be careful when applying cold water to the breasts. Only douche the tips of the nipples quickly. Prolonged washing of the breasts could chill the mammary glands deeply causing bronchitis. Many women use ice to rub over the tips of the breasts. The intense cold causes a very strong static contraction in the mammary muscles without giving the time to cause a chill.
9. **Herbal bath:** Lavender, hyssop, mint, borage, yarrow, rosemary and chamomile are useful herbs for the skin used in bath water either separately or in a mixture.
10. **Milk bath:** It is an excellent recipe for the skin. Add a handful of powdered milk to the bath water.
11 **Vinegar bath:** This is very useful for an itchy or dry skin. Add a cup of vinegar to the bath water.
12. **Honey bath:** To leave the body skin feeling smooth and satiny, add a teaspoon of honey to your bath water.
13. **Oil bath:** Add almond or olive or sunflower oil to your bath water. Baby oil or mineral oil is not suitable as it cannot be absorbed by the skin.
14. **Bubble bath:** Mix and beat one egg, half cup shampoo and one teaspoon gelatine. Add the mixture to the bath water when the tap is running.

15. **Salt bath:** Mix two cups of ordinary washing soda, two tablespoons of potassium carbonate and four to five drops of aromatic oil (pine or lavender oil). Use a tablespoon of this mixture in a bucket of bath water.

16. **Starchy bath:** Mix a few tablespoons of laundry starch and a teaspoon of glycerine to your bath water. It will leave your skin beautifully smooth, tight and soft.

17. **Oatmeal or Bran bath:** Put one tablespoon of oatmeal in bath water. Oatmeal and bran contain oils and vegetable hormones which soothe and soften the skin.

18. **Milk and honey bath:** Collect the following ingredients:

    Two eggs
    ¼ cup of both almond and sunflower oil
    ½ cup of olive oil
    1 teaspoon honey
    2 teaspoons washing detergent
    ¼ cup of vodka
    ½ cup of milk

    Completely blend the eggs, honey and oils together. Now add to it the detergent. Continue beating and mix the vodka and milk which will make the oil slightly thinner and luxurious. Finally, add a few drops of perfume to it. This bath oil, when mixed to the bath water, leaves the skin feeling smooth, satiny and thoroughly pampered.

19. **A luxury bath:** To take bath, pour scented bath oil or bubble bath in the tub and run the tap. In the morning, prefer to take your bath under the shower. Cold water closes the skin pores and helps you shake off the early morning sluggishness.

    Remove the face make-up, if any with a cleansing lotion. Undress and tuck your hair away from your face and neck. Get into the bath tub, relax for a few minutes completely, apply soap to the upper part of your body and rub every part except your breast (in case of women) with friction mitt. Pay particular attention to your neck, which is the most neglected part of the body. Use a bath brush to clean the back of your body. Step out of the tub and towel your body dry by patting and rubbing it very gently. Apply talcum powder on the underarms, feet and pubic area. Rub body lotion or massage cream on the rest of your body. After a bath, relax for a few minutes.

20. **Sun bath:** A sun bath clears the skin of acne, heals mild infections, cleanses oily skin, gives a lovely tan and revives the whole body. On the other hand, a hot sun bath can wither a dry skin, burn a delicate one, distend the veins and cause burns and also a sun stroke. Sun bathing should vary from five to fifteen minutes. Never expose yourself to strong sun rays for more than 30 minutes at a time. To enjoy the beneficial effects of the sun is to play, walk or swim in the sunlight.

21. **Turkish bath:** Air is heated in a chamber having temperature of around 43–54°C or the patient is made to sit in a hot room having temperatures between 65.5–76.5°C. Then a plunge bath is given in a cooling room. The body is then given friction to knead the muscles and finally, given a shampoo. The patient is then rubbed for one

to two minutes. To induce perspiration, a hot foot bath or a hot fomentation is given to the spine. When the patient begins to perspire, he or she should enter the shampoo room. Rubbing and stroking are continued until the skin is smooth and polished. A Turkish bath helps in slimming and cures many chronic skin diseases. It is seen that patients lose 800 gms or more in a single bath session.

22. **Hot air bath:** It consists of exposure of the entire undressed body (with the exception of the head) to a superheated atmosphere having temperature from 48–82°C. It may precede a cold douche, a cold wet pack, a cold immersion, a cold sponge or a wet sheet rub following a hot bath to increase the tonus of blood vessels and energise the nerve centre of the skin. The hot air bath should be avoided in case of skin disorders, cardiac weakness, in case of diabetes and in advanced cases of nephritis.
23. **Graduated bath:** It is a full bath treatment. The patient should be rubbed continuously to produce a chilly sensation. The bath is administered every three hours to stimulate the nerves which makes the skin healthy and glowing. Avoid a very cold bath. A person suffering from heart disease should avoid this bath. Rub a cold towel after the bath.

Precautions while taking a therapeutic bath

- Avoid bath within three hours after a meal and one hour before it.
- Avoid hip bath and foot bath, two hours after a meal.
- Use clean and pure water for bathing.
- Strictly observe the temperature of the water and the duration of the bath for the desired effects.
- Women patients should not take any bath during menstruation. However, pregnant women can take only a hip bath till the completion of the third month.

Genital bath

Genital bath is very essential for the cleanliness of the genital organs. Sit on a stool in the tub. The water should be cold in summer. The water level in the tub should be one inch above the stool. Take a piece of cloth, dip it in water and gently rub your abdomen for two minutes. Then take hold of the foreskin of your penis in two fingers and rub it lightly with a soft piece of cloth, dipping in water often. Continue for ten minutes. Now rub the entire spine with wet towel for two minutes.

Women should rub their abdomen. Then take a piece of soft cloth, pull up the lips of the vagina and rub slowly. In the end, they should also rub their spine as above. No genital bath should be taken at the time of menstruation.

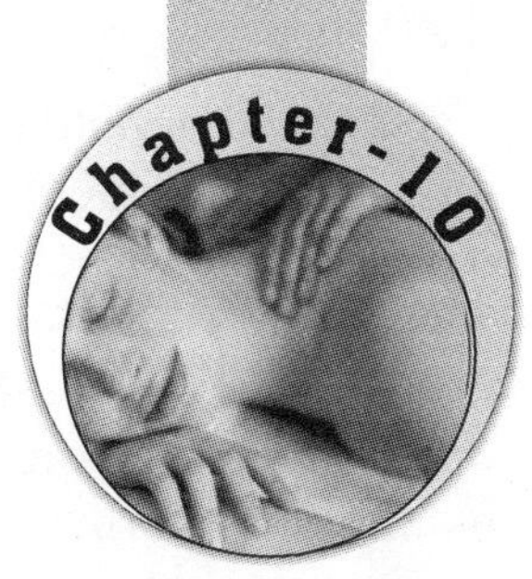

Massage Therapy

Physiological effects of massage

To obtain proper results from a scalp or facial massage, have a thorough knowledge of all the structures involved: the muscles, nerves and blood vessels. Every muscle and nerve has a motor point and the position of motor points will vary in location or individuals due to difference in body structures involved. Skilfully applied massage influences the structures and functions of the body, either directly or indirectly. The part of the body being massaged responds by a more active circulation, secretion, nutrition and excretion having the following beneficial results:

- The skin and all its structures are nourished.
- Fat cells in the subcutaneous tissue are reduced.
- The skin is rendered soft and pliable.
- The circulation of the blood is increased.
- The activity of the skin glands is stimulated.
- The muscle fibre is strengthened.
- The nerves are soothed and rested.
- Relieves pain.

Do's and Don'ts: Massage should not be done when certain conditions such as heart disorder, high blood pressure, inflamed and swollen joint, glandular swelling, a skin disease and broken capillaries exist. Massage calls for a firm, sure touch with strong flexible hands, self-control and quiet temperament. The hands should be kept soft by the use of cream, oils and lotions. The nails should be trimmed to prevent scratching of the skin. The palms should be warm and dry.

Reflexology and Relaxation

It is a 75-minute treatment in which finger pressure is applied to the reflex zones of the feet to stimulate the internal organs and systems of the body, helping to activate the body's natural healing ability and to restore balance. Afterwards, a relaxing massage promotes the further release of tension in the nervous and muscular systems, resulting in a deep state of relaxation and rest. Reflexology in the neck and head is a 30-minute treatment focussed on the zones of the head and the neck. It produces a decongestive effect, stimulates blood circulation, reduces inflammation, lowers the blood pressure; ideal for alleviating migraine and headaches. It is highly relaxing and strongly recommended for eliminating stress. Relaxing massage is a special 50-minute treatment for relieving accumulated stress, reducing muscle fatigue and improving the blood circulation.

Therapeutic massage

It is ideal for the treatment of sensitive areas affected by muscular tension, stress and fatigue. *Sports massage* is another 50-minute treatment before or after sports activities. It helps to maximise performance potential, reduces muscle fatigue, and eliminates toxins produced in the muscles during a physical exercise.

Anti-cellulite massage

A reductive massage that works on the zones with the highest concentrations of cellulite. Special movements are used to generate heat to help dissolve the body fat. Ideally, it should be followed with a *sauna session* and completed with a *shower house treatment.*

Lymphatic drainage

A massage therapy technique that helps to detoxify the skin and promotes its renewal. Helps to drain toxins and prevents premature ageing.

Shiatsu massage

In Japanese, *Shi* means finger, and *atsu* means pressure. The massage movement in which the fingers, palms and sometimes elbows are used to exercise pressure on specific points of the body to stimulate the energy channels and the internal organs. It reduces stress, alleviates aches, pains, fatigue, and the symptoms of a variety of diseases.

Ultrasonic massage

This provides a glow to the skin, improves blood circulation, activates sebaceous glands, improves dry skin and is especially effective for a dull and sallow skin. It works through an electric device. It is a highly effective massage treatment in deep penetration of the skin, very beneficial to do in winter.

Suction massage

This massage therapy can suck out the infection, unfriendly bacteria, dirt, dust, germs from the upper layer of the epidermis, from the deeper stratum in order to treat the secretions from the root. This *electric therapy* is totally safe, which is performed by the compressor. The

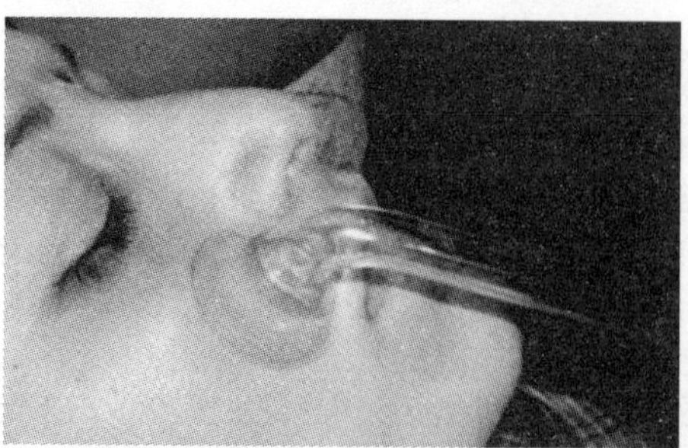

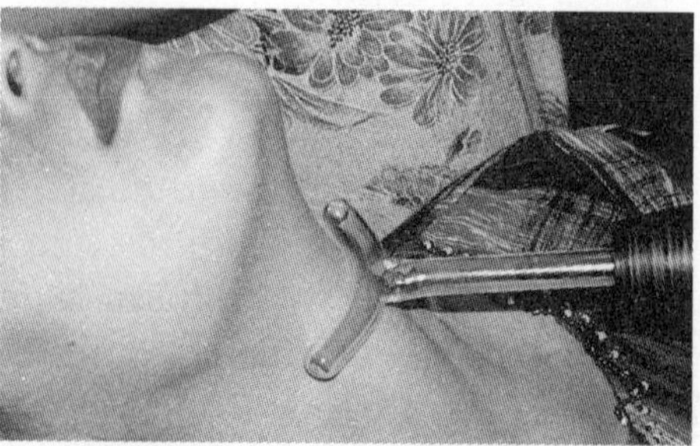

benefits include tightening of the skin; leaves skin germ free, helps in controlling sebum, improves blood circulation and removes infection.

Massage techniques

- Remove a little cleansing cream from the jar and blend it with the fingers to soften it. Using both hands apply the cream over the face.
- Start at the chin and with a sweeping movement, slide to the end of the jaw, from the base of the nose to the temple, along the side of the nose, between the brows and across the forehead to the temples.
- Take some additional cream, blend it, smooth down (optional movement) the neck, chest and the back.
- Start massaging at the centre of the forehead, move lightly around the eyes, then towards the temples and back to the centre of your forehead. Slide down the nose to the upper lip, smooth to the temples and the forehead, then move lightly down to the chin and finally, slide up towards your jawline, temples and your forehead.
- Remove the cream with cleansing tissues or a warm moist towel.
- Emollient (tissue) cream, selected according to the type of the skin, should be applied in the same manner as the cleansing cream on face, neck, shoulders and the chest. Use lanolin or hormone cream for dry skin and cold cream for an oily skin.

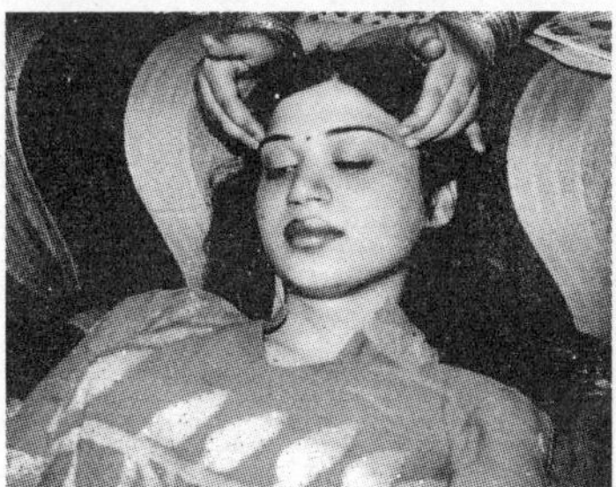
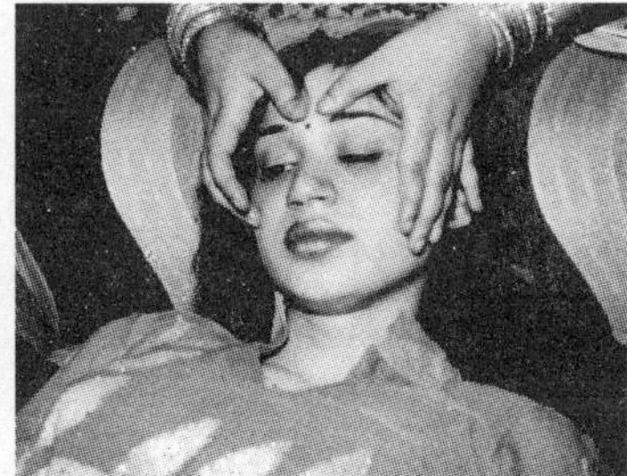
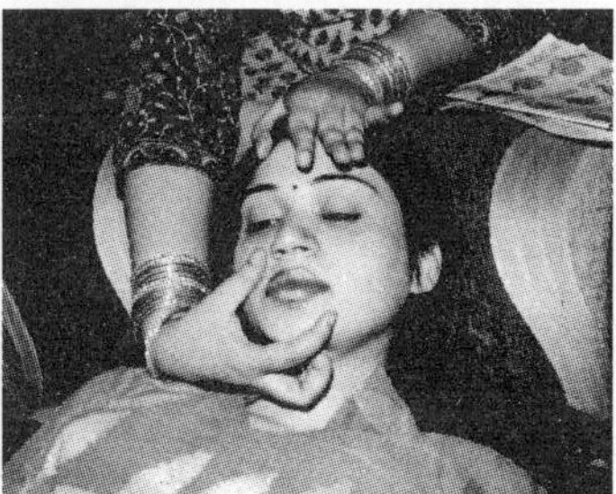

- Apply emollient (tissue) cream to your face, neck, shoulders and the chest. Apply an eye cream around the eyes and muscle oil around the neck.
- Massage the face, give manipulations using the hands (slightly cupped) and fingers. Start under the lower lip, press outwards in a continuous line with two fingers. Repeat several times. Pinch gently along the jawline, working outwards towards the ears.

What is lymphatic massage

In the human body, the heart is on the left-hand side and our lymphatic duct is on the right-hand side. This helps in purifying the blood from the heart. There are 18 lymphatic nodes in our body. The lymphatic massage has the following advantages:

- Waste products from our body are removed by opening up the lymphatic nodes.
- Removes wastage from tissue and it helps in fighting infections.
- Improves blood circulation.
- Removes waste products like oils, grease and bacteria from our body.
- Relaxes our nodes.

- The fluids get removed from the veins through urine.
- This massage is excellent for skin disorders such as acne.

Ways to do lymphatic massage or lymphatic drainage

Lymphatic massage is always given before a normal massage with the following procedure:

- Removal of make-up.
- Cleansing routine of the skin.
- Treatment through gadgets.
- Touch therapy.
- Effleurage therapy.

Precautions: The following precautions are necessary before a lymphatic massage:

- Lie down absolutely straight before starting the massage.
- Persons below 16 years of age should not be given a lymphatic massage.
- Massage done in a wrong process sometimes leads to vomiting and headache.

Motor points

In order to obtain maximum benefits from the facial massage, a thorough knowledge of the motor nerve points that affect the underlying muscles of the face and neck is very essential. The location of the motor points varies among individuals due to difference in body structures. Motor points are used for face lifting. For the treatment, face lifting and toning machines are used on the motor points. This machine has two rods through which electric current is produced. These rods are used on the motor points, which help in tightening and lifting of the skin and bring it back to its actual position. The electric current so produced is adjusted according to the condition. The massage is not given directly on the skin. One should always lift the motor points after applying the treatment cream.

Important pressure points on the face

There are several reflex points on the face. Pressing these points helps to improve the blood circulation and energy flow in the face and also tones the skin. Hold each point for five seconds. These points are situated on the face, hands and feet and also on the other parts of the body.

- **If the face looks tired or is sagging :** Rub at the centre of the lower cheekbone at the outer corners of the eyes on both sides of the face.
- **In case of puffy eyes:** Rub on either side of the nose in line with the inner corners of the eyes.
- **If the face looks tired or is sagging:** Rub at the outer corners of the eyes on both the sides.
- **In case of droopy cheeks:** Rub the hollows just below the ears on both the sides of the face.
- **In case of eye bags and loose cheek muscles:** Rub the border line between the eye socket and the cheekbone on both sides of the face.
- **To tone up and energise the muscles of the entire body:** Rub at the centre of the palms of both the hands.

Various Massage Techniques to Fight Ageing

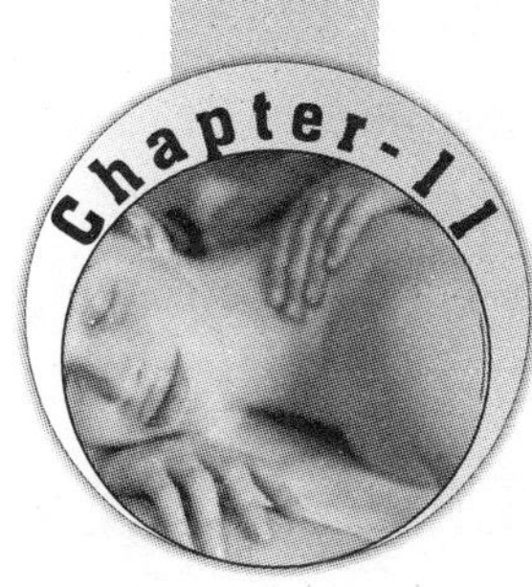

Thai massage

Traditional Thai Massage with its complete movements and stretch of every body muscle, is a unique combination of acupressure, breathing techniques, gentle stretches and healthy postures. This massage technique stimulates the flow of energy and balance is restored to the body—physically, emotionally, mentally and spiritually. This therapy ensures the following benefits:

- Releases strength and increases energy.
- Increases flexibility and range of motion.
- Provides deep relaxation pressure on feet and legs which is very soothing.
- Releases point of tension in the body which blocks the natural flow of energy.
- Helps homeostasis balance and harmony.
- Strengthens the internal organs.
- Promotes inner peace and a quiet mind.
- Assists alignment and postural integrity of the body.
- Suitable for postnatal mothers.
- Improves neurological functions.
- Treats muscular and general relaxation.
- Helps stress reduction.
- Relieves body pain and recovery from injury.
- Promotes circulation of the blood and lymph.
- Restores metabolic balance.

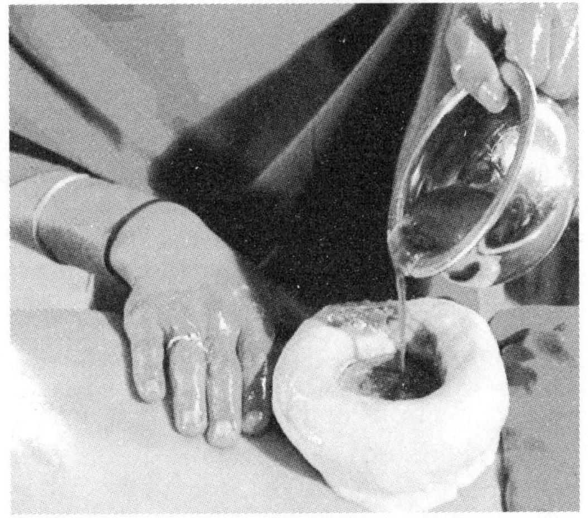

Panchkarma massage

Panchkarma Massage also known as *a touch of health,* relieves stress on muscles and internal organs. This therapeutic massage movement detoxifies the blockages inside the body and also beautifies the body giving a glow to the skin. It balances the body, mind and soul. Light and heavy movements and vigorous and gentle rhythmic and soothing movements are given on different body organs to achieve the maximum results.

Panchkarma Massage techniques are adopted according to the results the practitioner wants to achieve. They comprise vigorous to slow, simple to complex and hard to soft or gentle movements.

Chinese massage movement

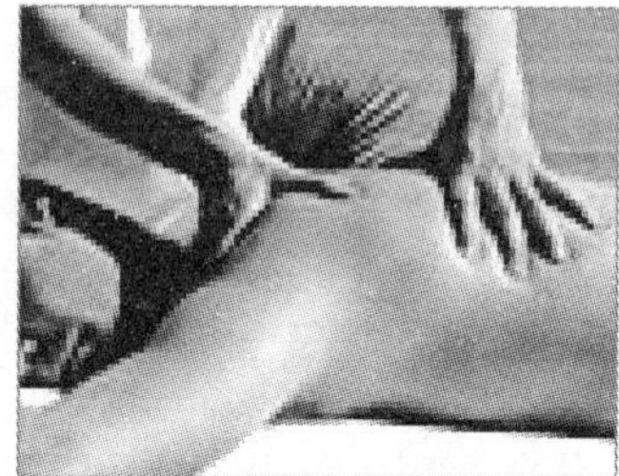

This massage movement is a medical practice and acupressure plays a major role in this, which energises and balances the body and mind. It is also beneficial in relieving pain, discomfort and many physiological imbalances.

Japanese massage system

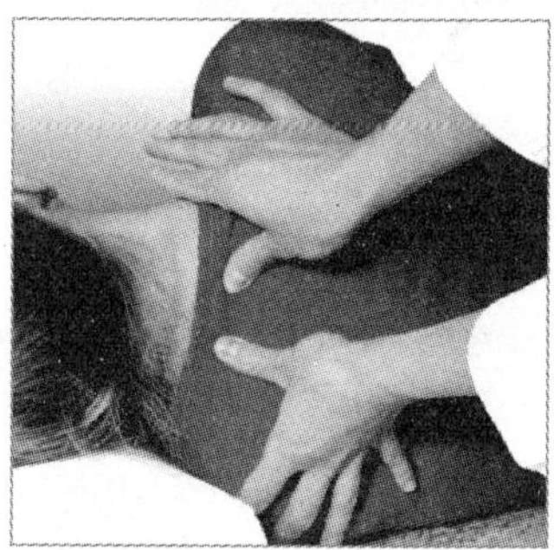

It is also called **Shiatsu** and is based on Oriental medical methods. According to this therapy, the human body has numerous points of energy, which can be described as energy points. By pressing these energy points, the energy level in our body increases. If we give proper and regular pressure on these points, we can regain our lost energy, which not only improves our mental health and body metabolism but can also treat physical disharmony, simultaneously.

Head massage

It is very important to provide mental relaxation and it stimulates the energy points located on our scalp. It provides a strong and in-depth effect. *Head massage* stimulates the blood circulation, supplies nutrition to each hair root, relieves mental stress, relaxes hair follicles, nourishes the scalp, stimulates the sebaceous glands to produce natural oils, adds natural sheen and health to the hair, cures shoulder tension, removes dandruff flakes, relieves mental tension if done on the sections and nape of the neck, and helps in the healthy growth of hair if done near the temples and sides of the scalp. It stimulates the roots of the hair and keeps the facial muscles strong.

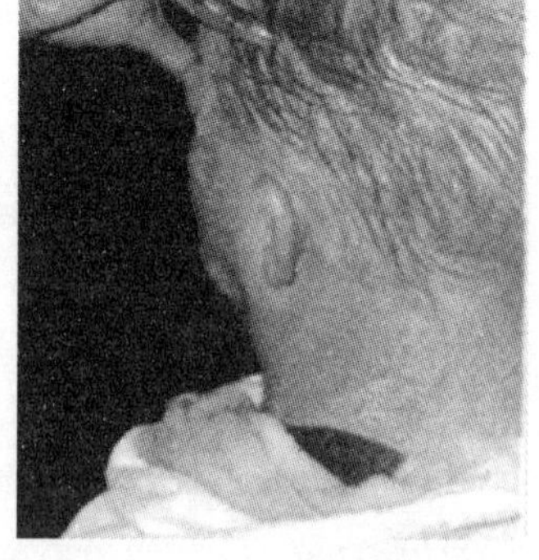

For a hair massage, cotton and oil (olive, coconut, mustard, almond, etc.) are required. The following steps ensure a good scalp massage:

- Remove jewellery and brush the hair.
- Section the hair about half inch. Dip the cotton into the oil and rub it all over the full length of each section of the scalp.

- Do scalp massage with five finger tip pressure. Do not exert heavy pressure. The fingers remain fixed to one part of the skin and the pressure moves the scalp. The various manipulations for scalp massage include *Effleurage, Petrissage, Friction, Vibration* and *Hacking* or *Tapotement.*

Effleurage

A massage manipulation used on the hairline by one or both hands or with pads of the thumb is known as effleurage. Apply pressure on various blood vessels. This movement leaves a relaxing, soothing, gentle, stroking and a circular effect. A massage is carried out with the pads of finger tips or palms of hands. It increases the blood circulation and strengthens the scalp tissues. This movement is useful for body massage too as it has a flowing and rhythmic effect with a constant pressure following through the venous flow of blood back to the heart. This movement aids relaxation, desquamation, blood circulation and strengthening of skin tissues.

Petrissage

It is a very important scalp manipulation, which involves light or heavy kneading, rolling, squeezing and pinching movements in circular motion to increase the blood circulation in the scalp. This massage movement is beneficial for the skin because it involves lifting the soft tissue away from the underlying structures. Use the palm of the hands, pads of fingers and thumbs while kneading, wringing and skin rolling.

It gives the following benefits:

- Softens and relaxes hard, contracted muscles.
- Eliminates fatigue.
- Stimulates sensory nerves.
- Increases blood circulation and lymph circulation.
- Helps to tone and strengthen the muscles of the skin.

Vibration

A rapid manipulation done with finger tips and palms. The massage can also be done with an **electrical vibrator**. It stimulates the nerves, relieves mental tension and increases blood circulation, cures all disorders of the scalp, makes the hair and the scalp soft and supple, cures baldness and gives shine and nutrition to the hair, etc. Vibration is a fine trembling movement for massaging the skin using pads of fingers and thumb and palms of the hand. The movement can be static or in the running form, always applied along a nerve path. It leaves the following effects on the skin:

- Stimulates the nerves.
- Loosens scar tissues and stretches adhesion.
- Relieves pain.

Hacking or tapotement

This movement consists of stroking the skin with the sides of the hands and partly with the flat finger tips. The movement is usually carried out with the hands freely swinging from the wrist. It helps increase in blood circulation. Avoid this massage movement when the person is suffering from high blood pressure and heart diseases. When applied on the skin, the movement involves striking the skin surface with alternate hands. The wrist has to be loose and mobile to produce a light springy movement, such as *cupping, pounding, pinching and hacking*. It has the following effects on the skin:

- Increases the blood circulation thus producing erythema.
- Strengthens and tones the muscles of the skin.
- Stimulates the sensory nerves.
- Increases lymph circulation.
- Redistributes fatty tissues.

Friction movement

Small circular movements produced by the pads of the fingers and thumbs are applied only on the skin to exert pressure. It gives the following benefits:

- Breaks down nodules and fibrous adhesion.
- Increases blood and lymph circulation.

Precautions while massaging the face

1. A massage is effective only if the skin is clean.
2. Wash hands with soap before massaging.
3. Remove all traces of make-up before massaging, otherwise the pores of the skin will be blocked by particles of stale make-up items.
4. If there are blackheads, remove them before massage.
5. If the skin is overdry, use moisturiser before the massage.
6. If the skin is too oily, remove the oiliness with cleansing milk, pH acid or fresh lemon juice.
7. Never massage over an area where redness, swelling or pus is present.
8. Do not break contact with the skin until the massage is finished.
9. Keep your fingernails short enough to avoid scratching on the skin.

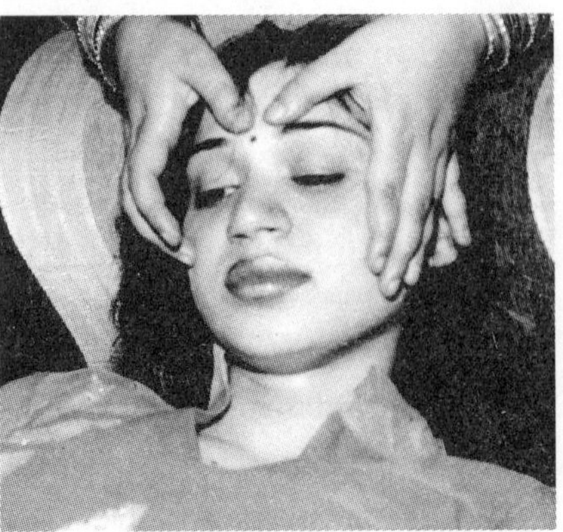

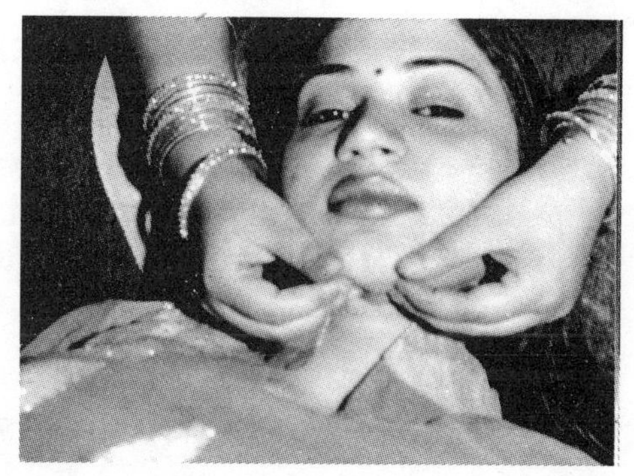

10. Always massage towards the origin of the muscles.
11. Do not press the delicate skin around the eyes.
12. Massage for a minimum of 15 to 20 minutes, as the cream takes that much time to get absorbed. Wipe off the extra cream with a cotton swab soaked in water.
13. Start the massage from the neck upwards and end at the forehead or temples because all the veins and tissues get a proper blood circulation by this process.
14. If the skin is damp, use astringent lotion before massage.
15. The best time for massage is before going to bed at night.
16. Use slimming cream for massage if the facial skin is fleshy.

Some do's and don'ts in massage

1. Keep the hands supple before massage. To do this, start with the hand exercises by holding and squeezing the rubber ball followed by relaxing the fingers repeatedly, of one hand and then the other.
2. Rotate and stretch each finger and the thumb in each direction one by one, pulling it gently by the other hand. Also press and hold the fingers against each other. The palms, however, should not touch.
3. A rhythmic massage sends waves of relaxation – throughout the body.
4. If you feel pain or are uncomfortable during the massage, inform the masseur.
5. Shape your hands to the contours of the body.
6. Vary pressure from very light to very strong when massaging. The pressure of the massage should be lighter over bony areas and firmer over the muscles. Do not apply heavy pressure when massaging.
7. Concentrate on the massage, aviod talking when massaging.
8. To give a good massage, be totally relaxed.
9. Do not worry if your initial movements seem clumsy. Practice makes one perfect.
10. Do not massage if suffering from:
    (i) An infection or a contagious disease of the skin.
    (ii) High temperature.
    (iii) A skin infection, bruises or acute inflammation.
    (iv) An inflammatory condition such as thrombosis or phlebitis.

How to use the massage oil

Do not pour the oil directly on the body. Pour about a teaspoon of oil into the palm of one hand. Rub the hands gently then stroke oil on the body. During massage, one hand should remain in contact with the body. Pour a little oil on the back of one hand, stroke slowly with this hand, continue stroking and place your free hand lightly on the top of the massaging hand. Stroke the oil on to the body from the back of your hand.

Techniques of body massage

The prominent body massage movements are as follows:

- **Stroking:** The rhythmic slow movements applied by the palms and finger tips of both hands are soothing whereas the brisk movements are stimulating, improve circulation, relax tense muscles and soothe the jangled nerves. This movement includes *Fan Stroking*—used on almost all areas of the body, *Circle Stroking*—for massaging in wide curves (circles), *Cat Stroking*—a smooth, continuous, soothing movement and *Thumb Stroking*—performed with just the thumbs.
- **Kneading:** A specialised movement for the fleshy areas of the body, thighs and shoulders. It relaxes the tense muscles, improves circulation, brings fresh blood on the surface and eliminates the waste products. Use plenty of oil for this massage movement. Basic kneading, wringing and light kneading are deeper movements of this form.
- **Pressure:** This movement releases tension in the muscles. It is especially beneficial for massaging the spine and around the shoulder region, using little oil.
- **Knuckling:** Small, circling strokes of this massage movement leave a ripping effect, especially on the shoulders, chest, palms and soles.
- **Percussion:** Brisk, bouncy movement, usually applied on fleshy and muscular areas of the body to stimulate the nerves. Do not apply this movement on bony areas, broken veins and bruises.
- **Cradling:** A warm, comforting massage movement with both hands.
- **Criss-cross movement:** A massage movement gliding across both the hands with fingers facing away.

Benefits of body massage

A body massage relaxes the muscles, lowers the stress levels, relieves pains, induces a blissful state, cures backaches and body pains, and softens the tense and knotted muscles. Slow and rhythmic muscle movements (massage) calm the nerves of the entire body whereas fast and brisk movements invigorate them.

Massage of body organs

Back massage

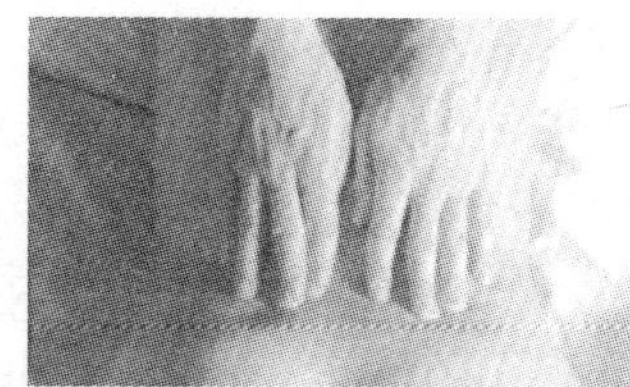

The spine is built of small bones called **vertebrae.** The **spinal cord** runs down through the spine in the back.

Massage Movements Used: Stroking movements, Fan Stroking and Kneading movements are applied from the base of neck and shoulders till our hands reach the waist.

The neck and shoulder massage

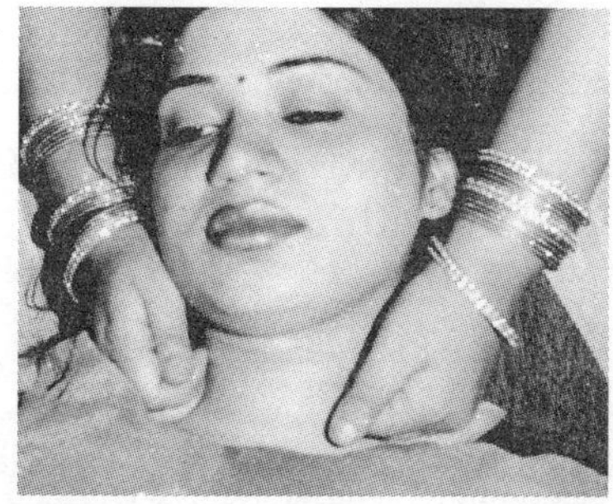

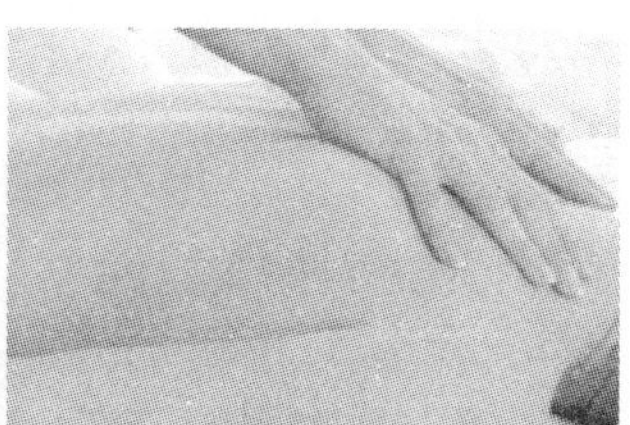

This region of the body has to support the weight of the head (5-7 kgs) and hence, such muscles remain tensed.

Massage Movements Used: Stroking, Kneading and Circular Pressure movements are applied to provide comfort and ease mental tension.

The buttocks massage

Tension also exists in the lower back and buttocks. Buttock muscles can be rid of tension through this massage.

Massage Movements Used: Circle Stroking, Fan Stroking and Pressure Movements.

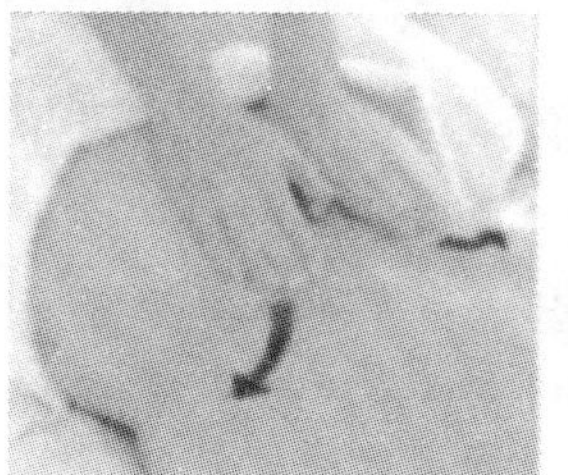

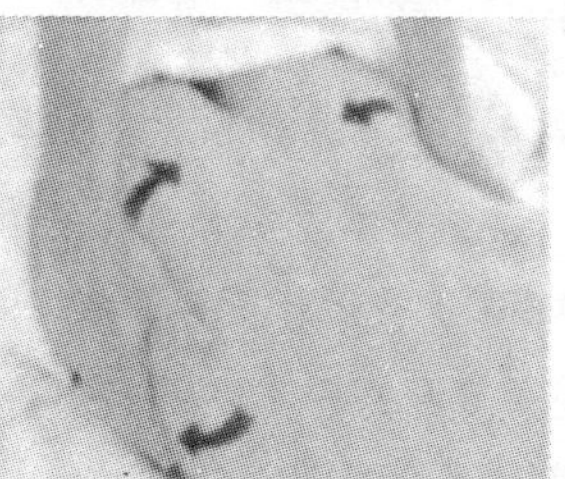

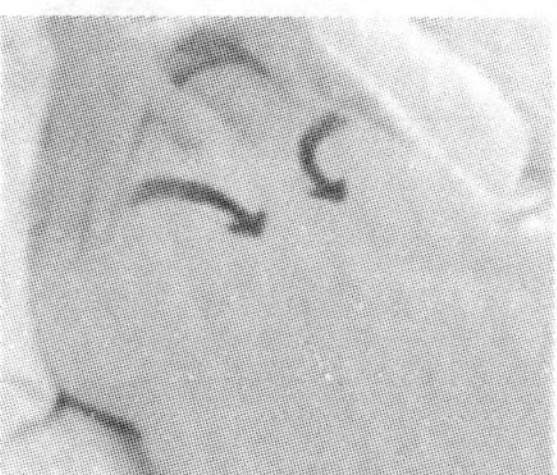

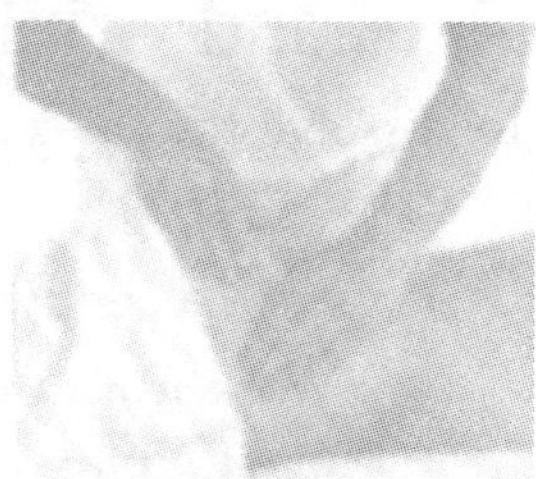

The spine massage

The spinal cord is a bunch of nerve fibres running down through the spine and are attached to the pelvis, mounted on the vertebrae.

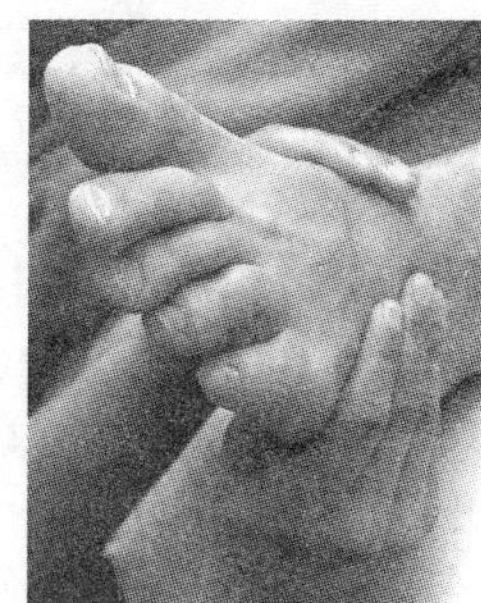

Massage Movements Used: Massage with the index and the middle finger simultaneously with both hands stroking downwards. Do no press hard on the vertebrae.

Foot massage

A foot massage not only relaxes thousands of nerve endings that exist in the sole but also refreshes and stimulates the whole body. The feet contain almost 25% of all the bones in the body. Each foot has 28 separate bones and muscles to support the body weight.

Massage Movements Used: Stroking, Thumb Stroking, Toe Massage, Pressure, Knuckling, Rotary Pressure, Hacking and Passive movements are applied in a foot massage.

Leg massage

Legs carry the weight of the entire body. These must be sturdy with strong bones. Massaging legs helps to reduce puffiness, swelling and aches.

Massage Movements Used: Stroking the legs, Kneading the calf, Stroking the calf, Criss-crossing the calf/thigh, Stroking thighs, Rotary Pressure Stroking, Passive movements and Massaging the back of legs are beneficial for the leg massage.

Arm massage

Tension and tiredness in the arms leads to headache, neck pain and arching shoulders.

Massage Movements Used: Apply Stroking and Fan Stroking movements, which alleviate many body disorders and are helpful in arm massage.

Abdomen Massage

Abdominal massage calms the nerves, stimulates the digestive system, cures a bad menstruation, helps in shedding flab and improves the skin texture.

Massage Movements Used: Stroking, Circle Stroking, Rotary Pressure movements, Kneading and Feather Stroking are important movements applied to shed off the extra weight, help drawing out tension, relaxing and also give a stimulating effect.

Lines and wrinkles under the eyes

To dissolve the lines and wrinkles under the eyes, the following massage movements should be tried:

- Stroke gently with the middle finger in circles around your eyes.
- Work from the bridge of your nose out over your eyebrows, pressing the temples.
- Pinch along your eyebrows from the centre to the temples.
- Press the bone under the eyebrows at the bridge of the nose with your thumb and the index finger.

Massage for expectant mothers

Careful, smooth and gentle massage movements benefit a woman during pregnancy (Do not forget to consult a doctor). Massage movements help to alleviate many complications such as tension, backache, insomnia and fatty deposits on the body. A pregnant woman should avoid deep pressures and percussion movements. A careful massage during the three trimesters of pregnancy and even before conception helps to increase the fertility of a woman.

Use all stroking techniques for the abdomen, back, shoulder and leg (and feet) massage. Remember, the massage strokes should be gentle and light. Use cushions under the shoulder, lower back and knees to reduce curves and discomfort. The massage done by a trained masseur makes childbirth easier. Lower back and shoulders are the areas which relieve tension while massaging. For the back massage, a pregnant woman should lie on her side or on a chair sitting or facing towards the back of the chair.

The following massage movements are recommended for a pregnant woman:

1. Gentle stroking on the abdomen with one hand following the other clockwise, stroking softly on the side of the waist upwards till both the hands reach the navel.
2. Cup your hands over the navel for a few seconds until you feel the heat, then lift your hands slowly.
3. Leg massage is especially beneficial as it soothes, relaxes and relieves the swelling and pain and cures the varicose veins and cramps in the legs, which are some of the common problems faced by expectant mothers.
    - Sleep wih the legs slightly raised above the level of the head. This posture relieves the swelling in the legs by draining the manual lymphatic system and purifies the body curing various skin diseases such as acne, eczema and dermatitis. Expectant women should undertake the abdominal massage after a strict advice of a doctor. Back massage cures backaches, morning sickness, etc., which are some of the common complaints during pregnancy. But avoid deep pressure to the lower back. Apply deep pressure in the centre of the sole towards the heel of the feet which helps in easy delivery and reduces the labour pain.

Massage after childbirth

A deep massage on the abdomen for about 40 days after delivery energises the mother, cures her body aches and brings the uterus back to its right position. To give an abdominal massage to a woman after childbirth, the following massage movements should be applied:

- Stroke the abdomen in all directions. Then gently knead across the abdomen in large clockwise circles. Start at the pubic bone applying a gentle pressure.
- Stroke slowly on the lower abdomen starting from the pubic bone to the navel. Cup your hands over the navel holding for a few seconds until you feel the heat accumulating under the hands. Then lift the hands slowly.

Treating cramps by massage

Women are often prone to cramps during and after an exercise or a massage. A cramped muscle lacks proper blood supply. Massage, however, improves the circulation of blood. To soothe cramps in the leg, lie on your back and raise the affected leg. Stroke the back of your thighs, followed by kneading and finally stroke the affected area.

In case of cramps in the calf, sit with the affected leg straight. Bend your foot up and stretch the calf muscles. Start kneading the muscles and you will feel relaxed. Finally, stroke the whole leg.

Massage treatment for weight loss

To overcome weight gain and reduce the extra flesh from the areas of the body such as the abdomen, thighs, buttocks and the waist, use the massage movements such as kneading, pummelling and stroking. Vigorous massage helps you to slim down. There are several techniques to fight the extra weight and obesity, as mentioned below:

1. Squeeze either side of the wrist above the wrist bones.
2. Press on the hollow inside the ankles just behind the bony prominence.
3. Press in the middle of the groove between the nose and the upper lip.

Massage alone cannot reduce weight or break down the fat. Weight-watchers should have control over their diet and undertake light exercises with massage. Remember, massage tones the skin, smoothes the body and produces energy by stimulating the blood circulation. Weight-watchers should concentrate on self-massage of the following fleshiest areas:

- **Abdomen:** Lie on your back and knead your abdomen thoroughly.
- **Hips:** Roll on the side, kneel and pummel your hips. Repeat on the other side.
- **Thighs:** Sit up and knead your thighs from the knee up to the hips.
- **Buttocks:** Pummel your thighs up to the buttocks.

Massage before and after exercising

Exercising tense muscles can badly damage them. Tense muscles do more work than what is required of them. They consume more oxygen and produce more wastes. Do a whole-body massage with stimulating movements to increase the blood supply before exercising. During exercise, waste products such as urea, acetic acid and carbolic acid are released into the muscles and the accumulation of such wastes cause stiffness and pain in the body. The lymphatic system, however, drains these wastes in a very slow process. A massage can speed up the elimination. A massage, firmly towards the heart with gentle stroking towards the lymph nodes can rejuvenate the heart. However, avoid massage on an injury. Just massage gently around it, kneading very gently. Do not massage around an open wound at all.

Drugless Therapies to Avoid Harmful Effects

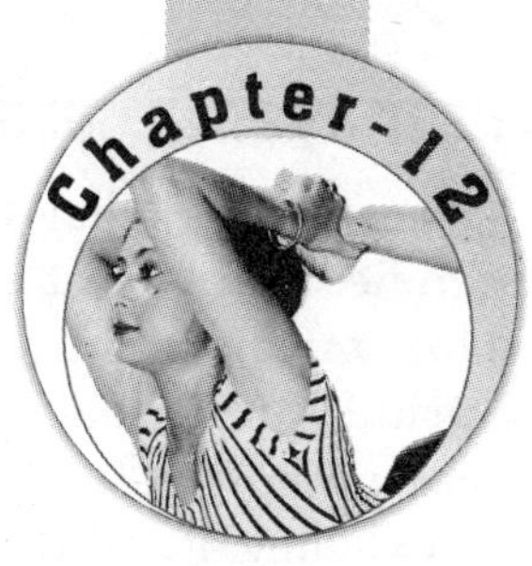

Depression, mental tension, insomnia and indigestion are the biggest enemies affecting the beauty of a human body. Depression is the most prevalent of all emotional disorders. An unpleasant experience a person has to endure due to the growing complexities of modern life and the resulting crisis, mental stress and strain in day-to-day living usually leads to this disorder.

The most striking symptoms of depression are:

- Feelings of acute sense.
- Sadness, giddiness and tiredness.
- Constipation and loss of appetite.
- Loss of energy, sleep disturbance, nightmares and repeated waking from midnight onwards.
- Low body temperature and blood pressure.
- Hot flushes and sensations of shivering.
- Loss of interest, itching, nausea, agitation and irritability.
- Aches and pains in the body, blurred vision and urine retention.
- Rapid loss of weight, frequent headaches and dizziness.

Depression is caused by the following:

- Depleted functioning of the adrenal glands.
- Irregular diet habits and digestive problems.
- Excessive use of drugs and intake of fats.

The following measures are taken to treat depression:

- Regulate the diet (exclude tea, coffee, alcohol, chocolate, cola, all white flour products, sugar, food colouring and strong condiments).
- Scientific relaxation and meditation.
- Yogic exercises, which produce chemical and psychological changes that improve mental health and change the hormone level in the blood. The following Yoga exercises are recommended.

Pranayama and meditation

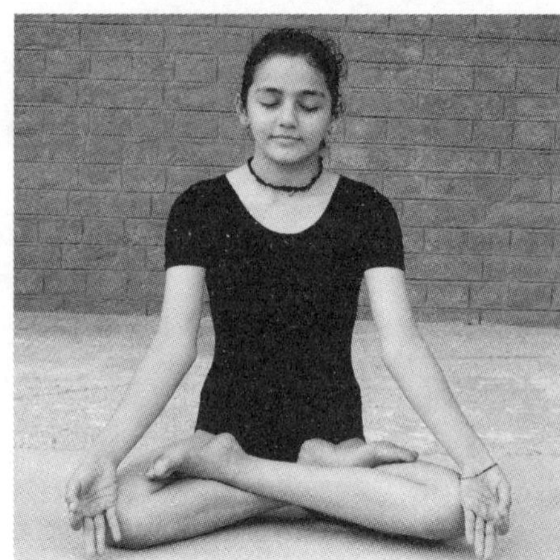

Prana means 'Vital Force' or 'Cosmic Energy' which signifies life or breath. *Yama* means control of the '*Prana*'. This means control of concentration and regular breathing essential to life. The cycle consists of the absorption of air by inhalation of oxygen and its expulsion by exhaling of carbonic gas. The yogic breathing consists of three parts as below:

1. **The Abdomen.**
2. **Thorax** (middle part of the chest)
3. **Clavicle** (upper part of the chest or collar bone)

Always inhale and exhale through the nose. The nose is to breathe, the mouth is to eat and to speak. On the whole, Pranayama means life and vice versa. A newborn baby starts breathing just after birth when the lungs are filled with air. However, before birth the baby is in the womb of the mother and it does not breathe but respiration still exists and oxygen is supplied to each cell of the growing baby inside the womb.

Meditation is a simple sitting posture. Sit with the left heel set against the perineum and the right heel on the left one. This posture supplies blood to the pelvic region and calms the nerves of the whole body.

Padmasana (lotus posture)

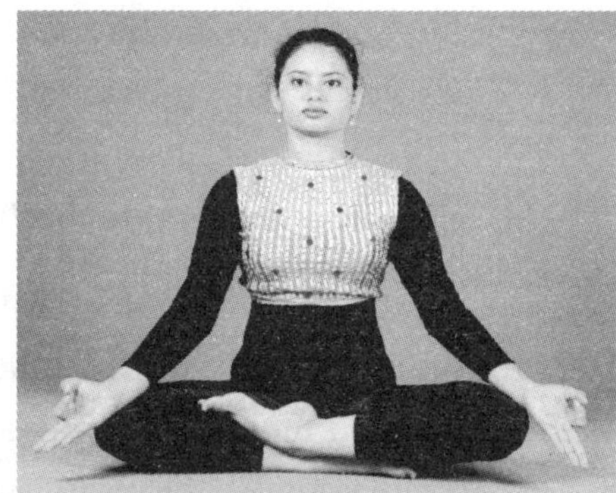

Keep the right foot on the left thigh and the left foot on the right thigh. Keep the hands on the knees, the back (spinal column) and the neck should be straight. *Padmasana* is described as a meditative posture having therapeutic advantages of developing physical and mental stability. It calms the nerves, relieves stiffness of the knees and joints, supplies blood to the abdominal region and the entire body is kept in complete equilibrium.

Dhanurasana (bow pose)

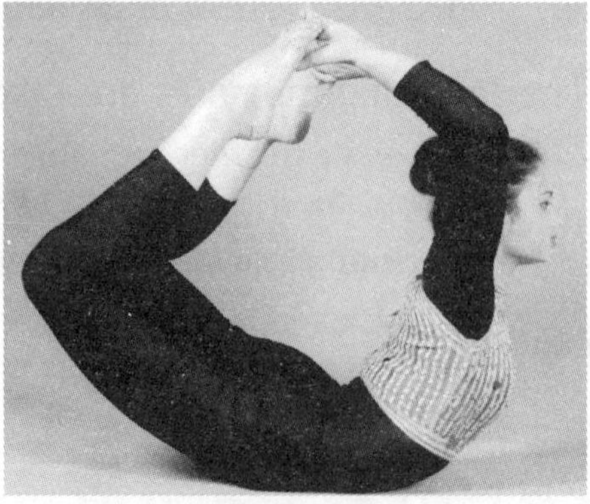

This *asana* is highly beneficial in the treatment of depression. To do this posture, lie on your stomach and keep your arms stretched on both the sides. Rest the chin on the ground and take the ankles in hands. Now raise the legs, head and upper part of the body while arching the back. Remain in this position as long as possible. This *asana* tones the abdominal organs, cures female disorders, stimulates endocrine glands and prevents fat formation around the stomach and hips.

Relaxation

There is a need to control our nervous system and mental emotional activities. Learn the art of scientific relaxation and meditation. Relaxation enables the muscles to work efficiently and eliminates fatigue by promoting blood circulation in the body. Practice of *Shavasana* (dead pose) creates a balance of the mind, the nervous system and the hormones. Thereby, it overcomes depression.

Shavasana (complete relaxation posture)

In Sanskrit, *Shava* means 'corpse' in which one lies on the back like a dead body with a relaxed mind. In this posture, keep your arms at the sides, legs stretched out slightly apart, eyes closed, breathe rhythmically, slowly and deeply, keeping the brain completely empty. This posture calms the heart and the nervous system. It cures high blood pressure, depression, eliminates the toxins accumulating in the blood, recharges your energy and regenerates the body cells.

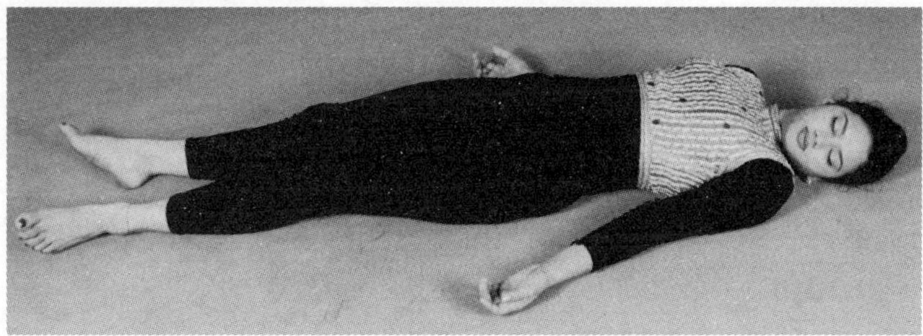

Sleep and insomnia

Sleep is Nature's greatest blessing of life which repairs the wear and tear of the body and mind. Most of the women sleep 45–60 minutes more than men. The amount of sleep required varies at different ages as mentioned below:

- Newborn : 18-20 hours
- Growing children : 10-12 hours
- Adults : 7-9 hours
- Aged persons : 5-7 hours

For good sleep, one should not sleep on one's back but on the side with both legs brought well up and the head and the shoulder slightly forward, in a well ventilated and hygienic room.

Insomnia deprives the person of mental rest. Sleeping on a bed that is neither too hard nor too soft but comfortable enough gives relief from tension and rejuvenates the brain and the body. The amount of sleep varies from individual to individual. Normally, seven to eight hours of sleep every night is adequate. The common causes of sleeplessness are mental tension, anxiety, worries, overwork, over-excitement, dull brain, anger and bitterness, constipation, dyspepsia, over-eating, excessive intake of tea or coffee, smoking, going to bed hungry, etc. Sleeping pills bring out indigestion, rashes on the skin, infection, circulatory and respiratory problems and mental confusion.

How to relieve insomnia

- Have a regular sleeping schedule. Early to bed at a fixed time, and early to rise is a good practice.
- Deficiency of key nutrients, especially vitamins and other chemicals, is the main cause of insomnia/which should be improved.
- A balanced diet and the eating pattern.
- Do not lie on your back, but on your side.
- Controlled breathing helps in inducing sleep.
- Have a regular exercise during the day. Exercise stimulates, eliminates lactic acid from the body, relieves stress and muscular tension and produces hormonal changes. Walking, jogging, skipping, cycling and swimming are ideal exercises.
- Application of hot spinal packs, hot fomentation to the spine and hot foot bath before retiring at night overcome insomnia.
- Yoga helps cure insomnia and tones up the whole body system. *Halasana* and *Sarvangasana* are recommended postures.

Halasana (plough posture)

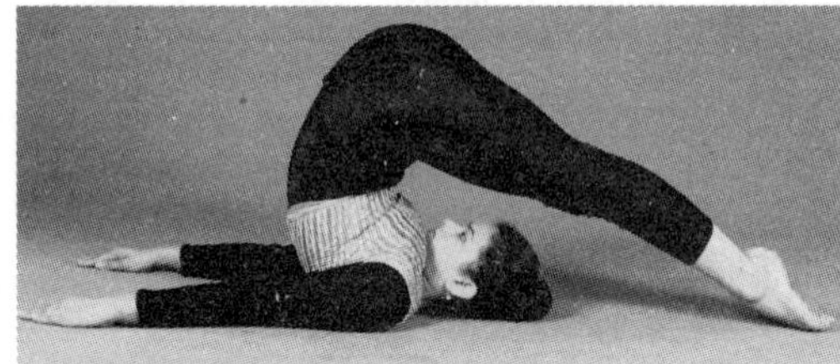

Lie flat on the back. Bring the heels and toes together. Stretch out the legs, raise them upwards, inhaling, till they reach vertical. Now start exhaling and lower the legs towards the head area, till the feet touch the floor. Remain in this position for 8-10 seconds and return to the starting position slowly. Repeat this posture for three to four times. This exercise has a good effect on the circulation of blood in the upper region of the body and restores a youthful look on the face.

Sarvangasana

Lie down on your back on the floor. Bring your heels and toes together and keep them loose. Start lifting both the legs together towards the ceiling, inhaling. Bring both the palms under the hips and raise the body upwards, pushing with both the hands. Exhale and keep both the palms on the side of the back for support. Stay in this position for 10-15 seconds. After standing on the shoulder for the desired time return to the ground. Rest and repeat the exercise for three to four times.

This *asana* supplies blood to the facial tissues, strengthens the digestive system, relieves abdominal troubles and energises the sex glands.

The sun looks white, but it has seven colours: *Violet, indigo, blue, green, yellow, orange and red,* out of which, violet, indigo and blue colours create a cool effect on the body, whereas yellow, orange and red colours create heat. *The remaining green colour is neutral.* The effect of different colours on various skin diseases is as below:

Colours	**Cure**
Violet	Baldness.
Indigo	Facial paralysis, indigestion, nervousness.
Blue	Mental depression, insomnia, nervous problem.
Green	Good for the eyes and improves eyesight.
Yellow	Indigestion, leprosy, diabetes.
Orange	Gout, mental nervousness and kidney problem.
Red	Anaemia, paralysis, leucoderma (white spots).

Have sun rays of the desired colour for 90 minutes after the sunrise and 60 minutes before sunset. Keep the glass of the desired colour in the sunlight in such a way that the rays fall on the affected area. If the sunlight is not possible, take a 100 watt coloured bulb or wrap coloured gelatin paper around a white bulb.

Coloured medicated water can also be given to the patient at an interval of 15 minutes to two hours, depending upon the intensity of the disease. Have a glass bottle of the desired colour or wrap gelatin paper of the desired colour on the white glass bottle. Fill in $^3/_4$th of the glass bottle of the desired colour and keep in the sunlight for at least three hours between 10 a.m. and 3 p.m.

Juice therapy

It is also known as Juice Fasting and is very effective to restore health and treat skin disorders as described below:

Disorder	**Recommended Juice**
Acne and Pimples	Carrot, cucumber, grapes, pear, potato, plum, spinach and tomato.
Anaemia	Apricot, strawberry, red grapes, beetroot, carrot, spinach and celery.
Skin Allergy	Apricot, beetroot, carrot, grapes and spinach.
Constipation	Apple, beetroot, carrot, grapes, lemon, pear, spinach and watercress.
Diarrhoea	Carrot, celery, lemon, papaya and pineapple.
Eczema	Beetroot, carrot, cucumber, red grapes and spinach.
Gout	Cucumber, cherry, pineapple, spinach and tomato.

Halitosis (bad breath)	Apple, carrot, grapefruit, lemon, pineapple, spinach and tomato.
Insomnia	Apple, carrot, celery, grapes, lemon and lettuce.
Neuritis (inflammation of nerves)	Apple, beetroot, carrot, orange and pineapple.
Obesity	Cherry, cabbage, carrot, grapefruit, lemon, orange and pineapple.
Psoriasis	Beetroot, carrot, cucumber and grapes.
Varicose veins	Beetroot, carrot, grapes, orange, tomato and watercress.

The rejuvenating therapies

There are various special herbal oils and herbs that trigger changes in mind and organs of the body to bring a balance and harmony to the overall system. These herbs are called **adaptogens** and they provide nutritional support, balance and modify systems of the body. Adaptogens are credited with properties that help the body adapt to stress, achieve body balance, increase protein biosynthesis, elevate body enzyme synthesis, promote general endocrine synthesis, improve mental power, increase physical ability, fight free radicals and improve the specific resistance to various stressors like heat, cold and wind.

The following rejuvenating therapies help to increase beauty:

1. **Shirodhara:** A thin thread of warm oil is poured over the fore-head and scalp. *Shirodhara* calms the mind, pacifies *vata*, cleanses, calms and balances the nervous system, relieves stress and improves mental clarity. *Shirodhara* is usually repeated three to four times a week for optimal benefit.

   Shirodhara is a deep relaxation technique that helps in insomnia, depression, excessive mental or emotional stress and brings about a meditative bliss. The treatment is followed with a gentle head, neck and shoulder massage.

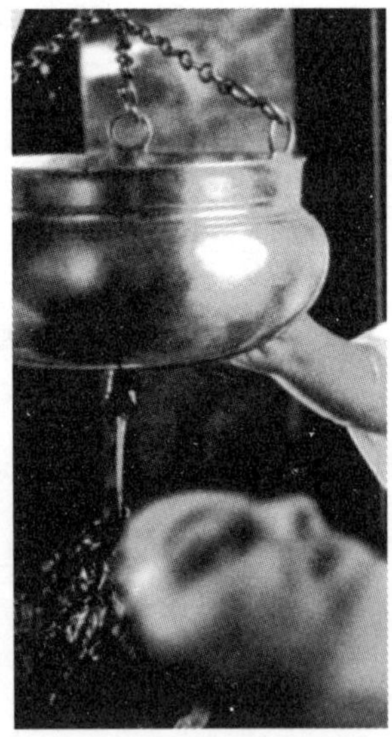

2. **Shirobasti:** Keeping oil on the head for about an hour in a leather cap is the technique of *shirobasti.* The patient sits on a comfortable chair wrapped in a blanket. Oil cooked with herbs is poured into the cap to cover the hair scalp. This treatment should be followed for 30 minutes to an hour depending upon the condition. Then gently massage the head, neck and shoulder.

   Shirobasti is an exotic and ancient process used to address several conditions, some of which include insomnia, chronic headaches, anxiety, hair loss, premature greying of hair, skin complexion and premature ageing.

3. **Nasya:** This is a procedure aimed at reducing the waste products from the head, throat and nose in the human body. *Nasya* is the introduction of medicated substances into the nose to stimulate secretion and remove impurities of the head and neck.

Nasya treatment is used in headaches, sinusitis, migraines, vascular headaches, nervousness, stiff neck, running eyes, ear infections, hearing loss, tinnitus, loss of smell and enhance beauty of the face. This treatment can be used several times a week in conjunction with other therapies like reflexology and head massage.

4. **Ampule Therapy:** It is a serum solution and fluids are penetrated into the deep stratums of the skin with the help of gadgets. They may be injected to a particular part of the skin with pure ampules under the guidance of an esthetician. This therapy provides instant results.
5. **Rasayanas:** *Rasayana* means to rejuvenate the body system and the tissues. It is a beneficial treatment for the face and scalp to encompass a head to toe beauty alongwith other treatments such as massage (*abhyanga*), steam (*svedana*), use of herbs, pastes and masks (*snehana*), foot reflexology, aromatherapy, colour therapy, gems and crystals, cleansing and strengthening *(panchkarma)* and rejuvenation *(kriya karma).* All these therapies and body treatments leave your skin looking and feeling fresh.
6. **Sidha Massage:** *Sidha Massage* promotes relaxation, calming of *vata*, *kapha* and *pitta.* It balances and increases the circulation of the body's largest organ: the skin. It also aids and facilitates the removal of waste products from the body. *Sidha Massage* increases lymph flow, strengthens the immune system and relieves muscle tension. This massage technique makes joints, ligaments and tendons mobile, thereby adding to the flexibility of the body organs besides helping to calm, relax, tone and balance the nervous system. It can be used to treat sleeplessness, regulates digestive and eliminative system, increases the production of collagen and elastin fibres, aids in the removal and prevention of wrinkles, and increases the suppleness of the skin.
7. **Abyanga:** This treatment is recommended for muscle soreness, joint pain and stiffness, nervousness, tension, stress, restlessness, lack of energy, immune dysfunction, fatigue, tiredness, paralysis/paresis of traumatic organ injury, poor digestion, poor elimination, sleeplessness and circulation of blood.
8. **Lymphatic Drainage Therapy:** This therapy needs gentle pressure on the lymphatic system to move the waste materials out of the body more quickly. This helps in controlling infections like acne, pimples and all the problems of the secreted skin type, resulting in clear skin internally as well as externally. The waste materials are drained out through urine.
9. **Seriatim Therapy:** This therapy is based on the conversation between client and technician through touch and senses. By this therapy, the emotions and mental activities of the patient are controlled and he feels relaxed. His mental tensions also get relieved.
10. **Sandalwood Treatment:** It is best suited for water retention, is diuretic and diaphoretic, leads to detoxification, stress-reduction, etc. Cellulite triggers skin to sweat and release toxins, and acts as a disinfectant. Sandalwood has been used for centuries in meditation and medicine. It promotes spiritual cleansing as well as cleansing the physical body. Sandalwood unlocks the trapped fluids and toxins that are stored in the tissues and is a disinfectant and astringent.

11. **Marine Therapy:** This therapy helps in uplifting the water level of the skin in the body. In this therapy, various nodes and modes are uplifted by pumping techniques and raising the water level which helps in delaying ageing and fine lines. It also controls dehydration and improves the lichen skin type.
12. **Panch Karma:** *Panch Karma* means '5 actions'. It is an ancient scientific system for detoxification and rejuvenates the whole system bringing youthfulness, strengthens the body and calms the mind. Traditionally, it is a preventive therapy aiming to clean the body and to eliminate the waste materials from the body.
13. **Shiatsu Therapy:** This therapy is also known as Acupressure. It is used to treat disorders by pressing various pressure points on the skin of the body. There are nearly 600 *Shiatsu Points* on the human body. Pressure on these points produces energy that flows in the body. To give treatment, the patient should lie on the floor with face down. Keep both the hands moving rhythmically along the meridians from one point to the other, pressing on each point for three to seven seconds. This therapy improves the circulation of blood and induces relaxation. The following steps are carried out to practise *Shiatsu*:
    - Pressing down either side of the spine.
    - Pressing down the buttocks and back of the legs with light pressure over the knees.
    - Pressing on the points on the arms, hands and front of the legs.
    - Pressing gently on all points on the abdomen in circles clockwise.
    - Pressing on the sole of the foot, in line with the big toe joint. This energises and stimulates the whole body.
    - Pressing on the front, one inch either side of the navel, reduces fat accumulated in the belly area. This stimulates and energises the abdominal area.
    - Pressing on the front, about three inches below the navel, helps weight reduction, cures cellulite and improves circulation.
    - Pressing on the front, four inches above the navel, energises the whole body.
    - Pressing on the back, about one inch above the waistline at two points, two inches away from the vertebrae.
    - Pressing on the back, at the waistline level on two points on either side of the vertebrae.
    - Pressing on the back, working up on either side of the vertebrae to the shoulder blades.
14. **Aromatherapy :** It is a technique to cure psychiatric disorders with essential oils, which have a therapeutic effect on the body as they are:
    - Analgesic
    - Antibiotic
    - Anti-fungal

- Anti-inflammatory
- Antioxidant
- Antiseptic
- Anti-spasmodic
- Antiviral
- Calment
- Carminative
- Depurative
- Digestive
- Diuretic
- Expectorant
- Hepatic
- Laxative
- Hypertensive and hypotensive
- Sedative
- Stimulant
- Toning and several other therapeutic effects.

Essential oils: Restore the balance of your emotions and mind, which:

- Soothe the nervous system and settle a worried mind.
- Calm anxiety and apprehension.
- Uplift depression.
- Improve concentration and memory.
- Pacify anger and frustration.

The effect of essential oils on skin: Essential oils penetrate deep into the layers of the skin. Due to their nourishing, cleansing and detoxifying qualities, these oils tighten the skin, increase the blood circulation, calm the nervous system and support the skin's functions. Essential oils should always be diluted into a steam bath, compress bath oil, body or skin lotions or massage oils. Choose appropriate essential oils for different types of skin.

- **Normal skin:** Chamomile, jasmine, geranium, neroli, rose, ylang ylang.
- **Oily skin:** Bergamot, cedarwood, cypress, lemon, geranium, sandalwood.
- **Dry skin:** Clary sage, lavender, jasmine, neroli, orange, vetiver.
- **Rough or broken skin:** Lavender, rose, chamomile, sandalwood.
- **Troubled skin:** Cedarwood, eucalyptus, peppermint, rosemary.
- **Broken veins:** Chamomile, lavender, neroli, rose, rosewood.

Therapeutic advantages of Aromatherapy are as follows:

- Improves blood circulation in the muscles, thereby reducing inflammation and pain.
- Promotes correct posture and helps to improve mobility.
- Improves the functioning of every internal organ of the body.
- Releases neck and shoulder tension and backache.
- Improves digestion, assimilation, elimination and cures constipation.
- Helps sprains, fractures, breaks and dislocations to heal promptly.
- Stimulates the immune system.
- Reduces high blood pressure.
- Helps cure headaches and migraines.
- Flushes the lymphatic system by mechanical elimination of harmful substances including toxins, bacteria and waste materials.
- Increases the efficiency and functioning of the kidneys.
- Encourages deep breathing.
- Relieves neuralgic, arthritic and rheumatic conditions.

15. **Treatment with essential oils:**

- **Atlas Cedar:** A woody aroma oil used in cosmetics and perfumes; relaxes tense muscles, calms emotions, helps breathing, eases pain and helps to stop hair loss (when blended with bergamot, cypress, ylang ylang, rosemary, juniper, vetiver, neroli, clary sage and frankincense).
- **Sweet Basil:** A slightly liquorice aroma which stimulates mental concentration, strengthens nervous system, revitalises the skin and has antiseptic properties (when blended with bergamot, clary sage and geranium).
- **Bay:** A powerful sweet, spicy herb which helps to stimulate hair growth, for relieving muscle spasms and strains, to improve the blood circulation and nervous exhaustion (when blended with citrus oils, rosemary, geranium, lavender and ylang ylang)
- **Bergamot:** A strong sweet spicy scent balances the nervous system, relieves anxiety and stress, has anti-viral properties and cures cold sores, eczema, psoriasis and postnatal

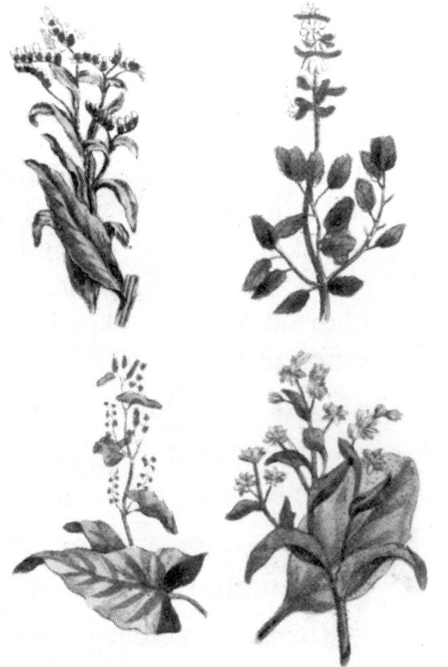

stress (when blended with lavender, neroli, jasmine, coriander, juniper, chamomile, lemon, geranium and cypress).

- **Black Pepper:** Warm peppery aroma having energising properties which helps increase the blood circulation, relieves muscle aches and stiffness (when blended with rosemary, lavender, frankincense, sandalwood and marjoram).
- **Chamomile:** A sweet and fruity aroma which relieves muscular pain, nervous tension, eases anxiety, relieves aches and pains, cures sunburn and skin rashes (when blended with bergamot, cypress, jasmine, juniper, neroli, frankincense, clary sage, vetiver, rosemary and ylang ylang.
- **Clary sage:** A spicy, hay-like aroma which helps to relieve stress and tension, eases pain, lifts melancholy, promotes restful sleep and is a powerful muscle relaxant (when blended with juniper, bergamot, lavender, frankincense, coriander, cardamom, geranium, sandalwood, cedarwood, pine and jasmine).
- **Coriander:** A spicy, sweet and fragrant aroma which helps in relieving muscular aches and pains, increasing circulation and curing nervous exhaustion (when blended with clary sage, ginger, bergamot, cypress, pine, jasmine, frankincense, neroli, sandalwood and citronella).
- **Fennel:** An earthy-peppery aroma capable of curing neuro-muscular spasms, rheumatism and arthritis, bronchitis, whooping cough, used to relieve stress, nervous tension, constipation and cellulitis (when blended with geranium, lavender, rose and sandalwood).
- **Frankincense:** A spicy, balsamic aroma which helps to calm, enhances meditation, elevates mind and spirit, helps breathing, cures skin trouble and scars and relieves mouth ulcers, boils, respiratory infections and impetigo (when blended with sandalwood, pine, vetiver, geranium, lavender, neroli, orange, bergamot and basil).
- **Geranium:** A leafy rose scent which helps to reduce stress and tension, ease pain, balance emotions and hormones; relieves fatigue and nervous exhaustion, lessens fluid retention and leaves the tonic effect on liver and kidneys (when blended with lavender, patchouli, clove, rose, neroli, sandalwood, jasmine, juniper and bergamot).
- **Ginger:** A warm spicy-woody odour which reduces muscular aches and pains, increases circulation, relieves bronchitis and nervous exhaustion and stimulates appetite (when blended with sandalwood, vetiver, patchouli, cedarwood, frankincense, coriander, rose, neroli and orange).
- **Grapefruit:** A fresh sweet citrus scent. It relieves muscle fatigue, used as an astringent for oily skin, refreshes and energises the body and stimulates detoxification (when blended with lemon, palmarosa, bergamot, neroli, rosemary, cardamom, geranium, lavender and cypress).
- **Jasmine:** A rich sweet scent which helps to relieve anxiety and nervous exhaustion, maintains healthy skin, relieves painful periods and labour pains (when blended with rose, sandalwood, clary sage and citrus oils).

- **Juniper:** A fresh pine-needle aroma which energises and relieves exhaustion, eases inflammation and spasms, improves mental clarity and memory, purifies and tones the body, cures cellulitis, cystitis, urinary tract infections and gout (when blended with vetiver, sandalwood, cedarwood, cypress, clary sage, pine, lavender, rosemary and geranium).
- **Lavender:** A sweet scent which relieves stress, tension and headache, promotes restful sleep, heals the skin, lowers high blood pressure and cures sunburn (when blended with cedarwood, clove, clary sage, pine, geranium, vetiver and patchouli).
- **Lemon:** A fresh lemon scent which balances the nervous system and purifies the body when blended with lavender, neroli, juniper, fennel, geranium, eucalyptus, chamomile, frankincense, sandalwood, rose and ylang ylang).

16. **Herbs that Heal the Skin**

Herbs	Properties	Skin care
Aloe Extract (*Gwarpatha*)	For softness, tenderness, moisturising, soothing calming.	For dry and sensitive skin, sunburn and skin irritation.
Aloe Vera	An emollient with hydrating, softening, healing, anti-microbial and anti-inflammatory properties.	Sunburn and sun exposed skin.
Arnica Extract	Antiseptic, astringent, anti-microbial, anticoagulant, anti-inflammatory.	Acne, reddened or tired skin.
Avocado oil	Bactericidal, soothing.	Used in bath oils, suntan preparations.
Balm	Calming, soothing, healing, anti-spasmodic, tightening and anti-bacterial in nature.	Eczema, dry skin, acne and blemishes.
Basil (*Tulsi*)	Stimulating, tonic, anti-bacterial, purifying and anti-microbial in nature.	Acne preparations.
Blackberry (*Jamun*)	Astringent and tonic, rich in vitamin C.	Scaly conditions, acne and psoriasis.
Birch (*Bhojpatra*)	Astringent, antiseptic, softening and stimulating in nature.	Acne, eczema, sunburn and hair loss.
Borage (*Pattharchoor*)	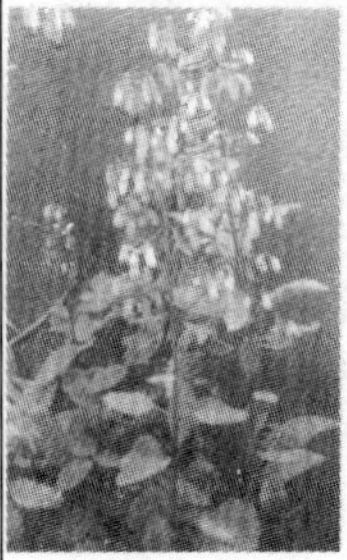 Anti-irritant and hydrating in nature.	Cures allergic reaction and ringworms.
Bergamot (*Zabir*)	Antiseptic, bacterial.	Oily skin, acne and seborrhoeic conditions.
Carrot Oil	Cleansing, depurative and draining.	Acne, dermatitis, skin rashes and wrinkles.
Calendula (*Genda*)	Healing, soothing, antiseptic, anti-itching, anti-inflammatory.	Eczema and spots.

Herbs	Properties	Skin care
Comfrey	Healing, astringent, emollient.	Itching, swelling, bruising, eczema, sunburn and cuts.
Cleavers (*Liptani ghas*)	Toning.	Dandruff, leprosy, eczema and skin cancers.
Clove (*Laung*)	Antiseptic, cicatrizant.	Skin tonic.
Chamomile (*Babuna ka paudha*)	Anti-allergic, healing, cooling, analgesic and antiseptic in nature.	Dermatitis, tumours, ulcers and used as a face wash.
Dandelion (*Kukraundha*)	Tonic, refreshing.	Pimples, acne, spots, inflamed skin, dry skin and corrects pH balance.
Elder	Astringent, antiseptic, cooling and emollient.	Sunburn, freckles, inflamed skin, dry skin and crow's feet.
Emblica (*Amla*)	Astringent, rich in Vitamin C.	Hair and skin.
Garlic (*Lehsun*)	Antiseptic, bactericide.	Acne, eczema and swelling.
Henna (*Mehendi*)	Astringent, antiseptic, cooling in nature.	Acne and eczema.
Horsetail Extract (*Equisetum ka paudha*)	Stimulating, astringent, soothing, healing and softening.	Acne, anti-ageing and wrinkles.
Hyssop Oil (*Zufah yabis*)	Healing, tonic, stimulating.	Cures dermatitis, eczema and wounds.
Jasmine Oil (*Chameli ka tel*)	Moisturising, soothing, healing.	Dermatitis, dry and sensitive skin.
Juniper Oil (*Habusha*)	Antiseptic, astringent, cleansing, toning.	Acne, eczema and dermatitis.
Lavender	Anti-allergic, anti-inflammatory, antiseptic, anti-bacterial, anti-spasmodic, balancing, antibacterial, energising, soothing healing and tonic, stimulating, etc.	Oily skin, acne, dermatitis, burn and psoriasis.
Lettuce (*Salad patta*)	Cooling effect.	Skin inflammation, sunburn and redness.
Marigold (*Genda*)	Antiseptic, healing and soothing in nature.	Sunburn, rashes, ulcers, varicose veins and oily skin.
Mint (*Pudina*)	Cooling, tonic, stimulating, antiseptic and relaxing, in nature.	Acne and dermatitis.
Myrrh (*Beejabol*)	Disinfectant, antiseptic, tonic, sedative, stimulant, astringent.	Acne, and used as a face mask.
Myrtle (*Vilayati Mehendi*).	Astringent, antiseptic in nature	To cure acne and oily skin.

Herbs	Properties	Skin care
Nettle (*Bichhoobuti*)	Anti-inflammatory, astringent, bacterial, healing, deodorant, antioxidant and stimulating in nature.	Eczema, sunburn.
Olive Oil (*Jaitun ka tel*)	Astringent, antiseptic, antioxidant, vasodilatant, etc.	Anti-ageing.
Rose (*Gulab*)	Astringent, tonic, deodorant, antiseptic, disinfectant, cleansing, moisturising, etc.	Dry and sensitive skin, lesions, wrinkles and aged skin.
Rosemary (*Rusmari*)	Astringent, toning, deodorant, antiseptic, re-activating, anti-bacterial, softening, and invigorating.	Tonic for skin and scalp, acne, dermatitis, skin regeneration and eczema.
Sage (*Safakuss*)	Depurative, healing, astringent, and invigorating.	Acne and oily skin.
Sandalwood	Astringent, anti-inflammatory, anti-bacterial, tonic, cooling, and soothing in nature.	Acne and oily skin.
Sesame Oil *(Til ka tel)*	Emollient	To cure suntan and used as a lotion.
Shikakai *(Kochi)*	Cleaning	Dandruff and skin.
Soap Nut *(Reetha)*	Cleaning	Pimples and scabies.
Strawberry	Astringent, cooling.	Eczema, pruritis and sunburn.
Tea Tree Oil	Antiseptic, germicidal, expectorant.	Seborrhoea, acne, psoriasis, eczema, dermatitis, itching and redness of skin.
Turmeric *(Haldi)*	Healing, tonic, stimulating, anti- inflammatory, softening and purifying.	Acne, eczema, burns, rashes, infection and ulcers.
Vervain	Curing, antiseptic.	Skin infections.
Walnut *(Akhrot)*	Soothing, astringent, anti-itching, fungistatic.	Sunburn, acne and skin diseases.
Witch-hazel (Hamamelis)	Anti-inflammatory, anti-itching, softening and healing emollient.	Burns, sunburns and skin irritation.
Yarrow *(Gandana)*	Astringent, antiseptic, anti-inflammatory, healing, calming.	Oily and acne skin.

17. **Magical *mudras* for beauty:**

Mudra No. 1 : ***Gyan Mudra***

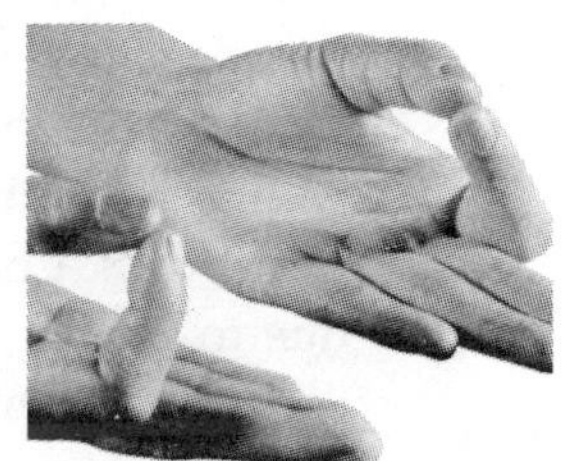

Touch the tip of the thumb with the tip of the index finger, keeping the remaining fingers straight. You can practise this *mudra* in meditation or in *Padmasana*. This *mudra* cures mental disorders, depression and sleeplessness—which is a healthy sign of hidden beauty. Practise it as long as possible.

Mudra No.2 : ***Prithvi Mudra***

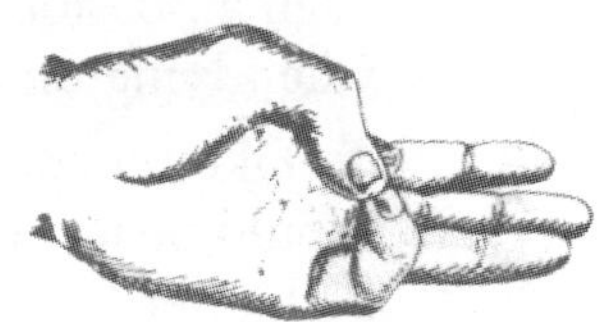

Press the tip of your ring finger with the tip of your thumb to overcome the physical weakness of the body. This *mudra* helps the weak persons to gain weight and increase the lustre of the skin and make it glowing.

Mudra No. 3 : ***Varun Mudra***

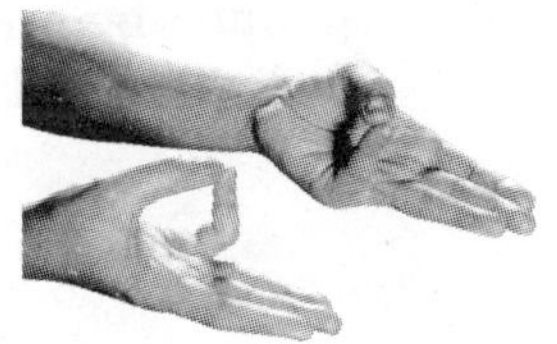

In this case, the tip of the thumb is pressed by the tip of the little finger. It helps to produce moisture in the body, the dry skin restores moisture and drains off impurities of the blood improving the skin texture, complexion and relieves pain due to cramps.

Mudra No. 4 : ***Vayu Mudra***

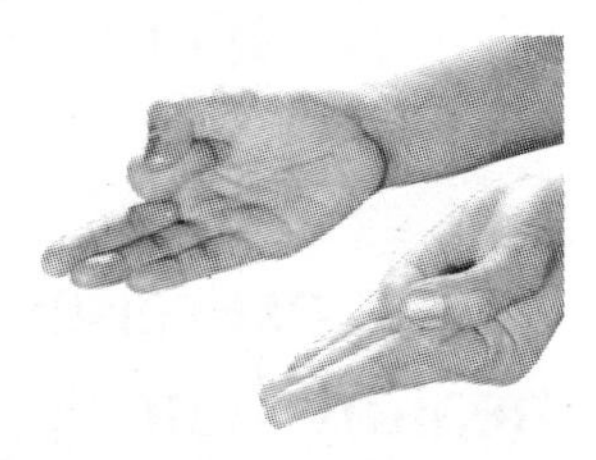

Press the side of the index finger with the tip of the thumb as shown in the illustration, practising for 30–45 minutes daily. This *mudra* helps to strengthen muscles of the body and brain, and cures rheumatism, gout, arthritis, trembling of nerves *(Parkinson's disease)*, palsy of face and stiff neck or cervical spondylosis.

Mudra No. 5 : ***Surya Mudra***

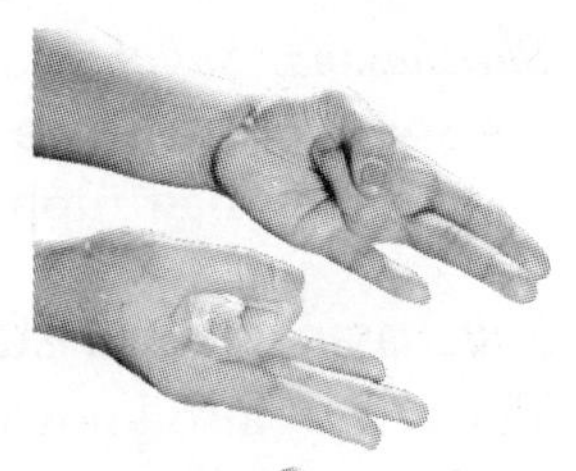

Bend the ring finger and press it with the tip of the thumb, preferably sitting in *Padmasana*. This *mudra* helps in reducing the body fat and mental tension. Practise this *mudra* for 10 to 15 minutes daily in the morning and in the evening.

Mudra No. 6: ***Jalodarnashak Mudra***

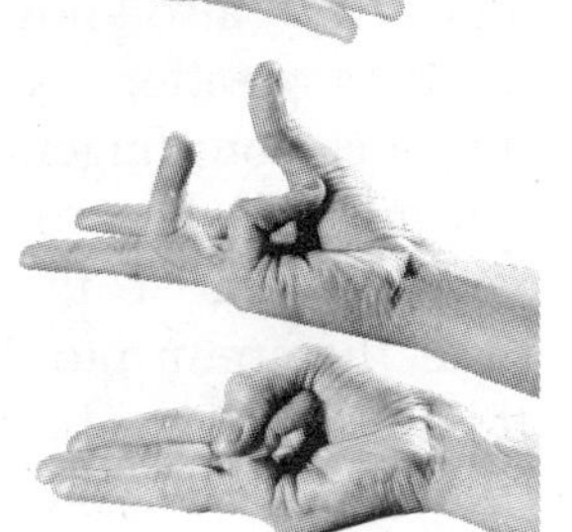

Bend you little finger to touch the base of your thumb and press it with the tip of your thumb keeping the rest of the three fringers straight. This *mudra* helps curing an over oily skin.

18. **Enema Therapy**

It is also known as **Rectal Irrigation** and is very beneficial for cleaning the bowel—a base of real beauty. An enema involves the injection of fluid into the rectum. Lukewarm water, with or without lime, (aproximately 1.5 litre) is used for cleaning the bowel. A hot water enema is beneficial in relieving irritation due to inflammation of the rectum and painful haemorrhoids or piles. Enema can help severe constipation and benefits women suffering from leucorrhoea (white discharge from the vagina), besides causing the skin to glow. Enema can be taken when lying on the floor or in standing position.

To take enema, lie down on a hard bed, the foot of the bed should be few inches higher than the bed. The buttocks should be higher than the rest of body. Facilitate the introduction of liquid through the rectum from the vessel containing hot water suspended at a height of 36 inches from the body. Let the water go into the rectum, retain it for two to three minutes before going to the toilet. Do not stain at the stools after an enema. Remember, a clean bowel plays a wonderful role in skin beauty.

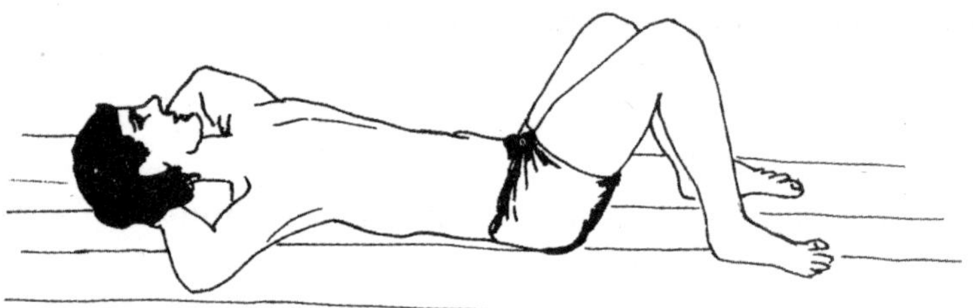

Yogic exercises for skin beauty and healthy hair

Shirshasana, Salamba Shirshasana, Ushtrasana and *Viparitakarani* are some of the Yoga postures recommended for skin beauty and healthy hair (upper part of the body).

Shirshasana (head stand posture)

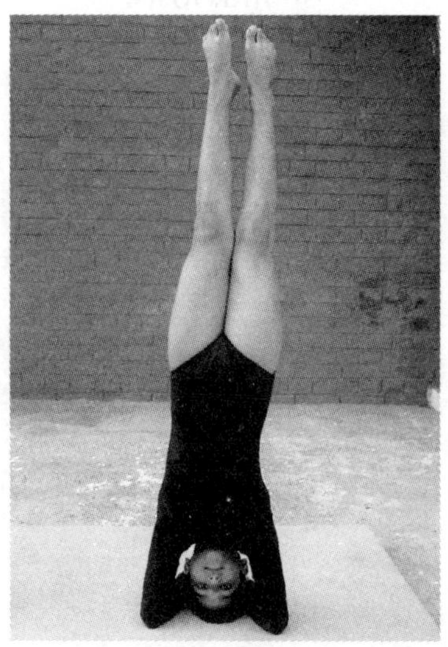

This *asana,* also known as the 'king of asanas', is performed in a sitting position. Kneel in front, resting your forearms and interlock your fingers on the head. Slowly raise your knees and the hips off the ground in steps till the straightened legs are perpendicular to the floor. Remain in this position for some time, then return to the initial position. If you are unable to do this posture in the beginning, practise the posture taking support of the wall. Lift your shoulders through your legs backward or forward slowly.

The therapeutic advantages of this *asana* include:

- Increased blood supply and blood circulation in the head and the upper part of body, which enhances your facial beauty and growth of hair.
- This *asana* removes fatigue, builds up energy, promotes growth and improves concentration and willpower.
- Has a beneficial effect on the endocrine and digestive systems.

Salamba shirshasana

The therapeutic advantages of this yogic exercise are similar to those of *Shirshasana.* The body is held straight, up-side down on the head. It promotes blood circulation and removes congestion of blood. To practise this *asana*, take the position of *Shirshasana* and bring both the legs horizontally parallel to the ground. This posture is extremely beneficial for disorders of the genito-urinary and reproductive organs.

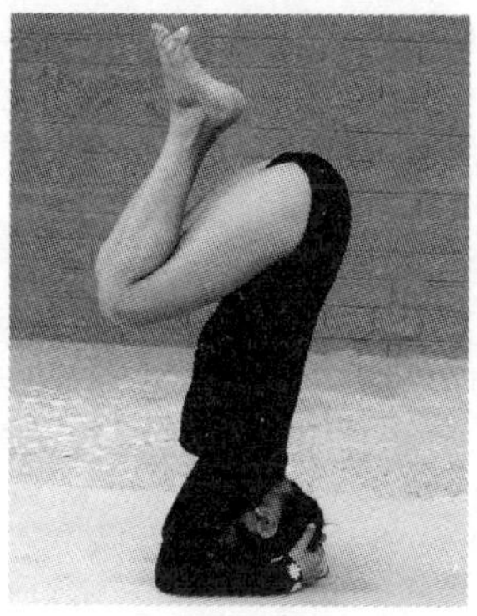

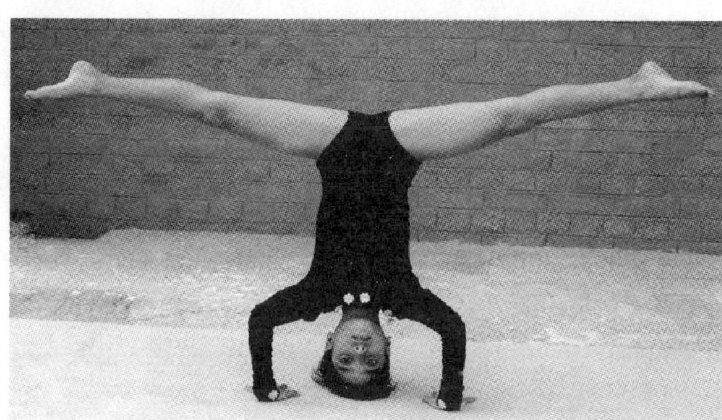

Ushtrasana (camel posture)

This *asana* helps remove stiffness in the neck and shoulders, cures visionary and voice defects, throat troubles, tonsils, chronic headaches and problems of the respiratory system. This *asana* activates the facial tissues and strengthens the muscles of the abdomen, thighs, chest and regenerates the kidneys.

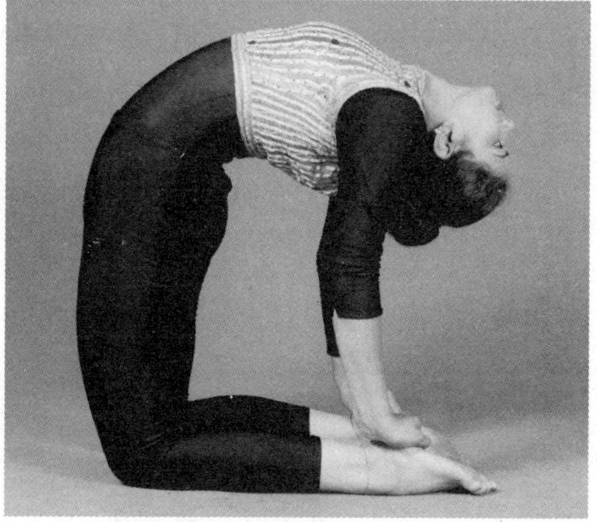

To practise this *asana*, fold the legs at your knees keeping them about six inches apart. Rest your hands on your hips and stand on your knees. Let the ankles and and the toes of both the legs fall flat on the floor. Curve back and catch hold of the soles of your feet. After 10-15 counts, return to the starting position. Repeat this exercise for three to four times.

Viparitakarani asana (inverted posture)

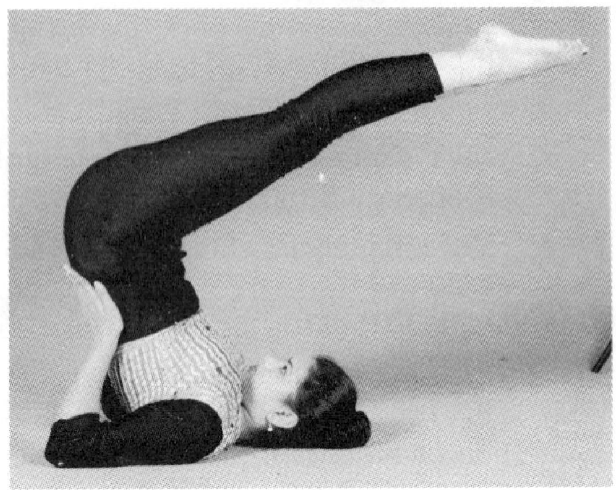

In Sanskrit, *Viparita* means 'Inverted' and *karani* means 'Action'. Lie on the back and inhale. Raise your legs and hips with the arms and exhale. The legs should form an angle of 60-70° with the ground. Now lower the legs gently to the ground. Relax for some time and repeat this two to three times. If you are suffering from blood pressure problems consult a doctor before performing this posture. The therapeutic advantages of this yogic posture include:

- Reviving the whole body.
- Preventing the formation of facial wrinkles.
- Increasing the flow of blood to the neck, throat and head.
- Regenerating the thyroid and pituitary glands, and the nervous system.

Slimming techniques

A healthy body is beautiful. A fat surplus of 8–15 percent over the normal weight must be considered as overweight. Beyond that, it is obesity. Over 30 percent, it is extreme obesity. Poor functioning of the digestive system, nervous factors, heredity factors, sedentary lifestyle and constipation are some of the prominent causes of overweight. There are **three categories of overweight :**

1. **Fatty Overweight:** Fat and muscle uniformly spread and more usual in male, often more noticeable over the upper part of body such as the head, neck, arms and trunk.
2. **Watery Overweight:** It does not affect the muscles and is most usual over the lower part of the body, common among the women.
3. **Cellulitis:** It is a form of infiltration rather than overweight.

The warning signals of overweight:

- The belt gets tight.
- There is strain on jacket buttons.
- The face starts growing round.
- The skin gets puffy.
- The skin loses its firmness and tautness.
- The shoulders get plump and hollows over the collar-bones.
- The fat overhangs the hips and the waist disappears.
- The buttocks enlarge.

- The girdle squeezes the flesh and swells out above and below it.
- The neck thickens and lose its normal contour.
- Double chin follows under the nape of the neck.
- Breasts sag down to the stomach.
- The stomach droops over the pubis.
- The pubis swells modestly over the genital organs.

It is observed that girls between the age of 14 and 18 tend to put on excess weight, largely because their bodies are undergoing natural changes around this time. To maintain a perfect figure, the amount of energy you consume must be equal to the amount of energy you burn. There is difference between obesity and overweight. Overweight is not obesity, but every obese person is overweight.

Recommended dietary allowance

The Recommended Dietary Allowance (RDA) suggests the major nutrients usually required by Indian men, women, working women, lactating mothers and women during pregnancy. An adult woman should consume aproximately 1900 to 2200 Kcal/day and an adult man should take about 2200 to 2500 Kcal/day as daily energy requirements. However, during pregnancy and breast feeding, the energy requirements are higher and a woman needs between 2200 to 2500 Kcal/day. These requirements should be supplemented by a balanced combination of carbohydrates, proteins, vegetables and fat moderation. The keyword here is quality and not quantity. It's not how much you eat, but what you eat. The following tips are suggested for a healthy nutritious diet. However, all food groups provide energy, which is expressed in technical terms as kilocalories (Kcal).

- **Proteins** (65 gms/day): This is required for good overall growth and development. Pulses, dairy products and soyabean are excellent sources of vegetarian protein. (Note gm = grams; mg = milligrams)
- **Calcium** (1000 mg/ day): This is required for the development of bones and teeth. Dairy products, soyabean products, green leafy vegetables and sesame seeds are loaded with calcium.
- **Iron** (40 mg/day): This is an essential component of haemoglobin that supplies oxygen to each cell of the human body (for the production of red blood cells). Foods with high iron sources are dried beans, cereals and pulses, dried fruits and green leafy vegetables.
- **Folic Acid** (400 mg/day): It is an essential vitamin, required especially by women going to conceive and also during the early stages of pregnancy for the growth and development of the foetus throughout the pregnancy and breast feeding period. Its deficiency leads to anaemia. Potatoes, vegetables, cereals and pulses, soyabean, nuts and sesame seeds are rich sources of folic acid.
- **Fat** (30 gms/day): This is also essential to enhance energy.

- **Vitamin C** (40 mg/day): This is necessary to fight against infections and diseases. It provides a structure to the bones, cartilage, muscles and blood vessels. Citrus fruits, *amla* and vegetables are rich sources of vitamin C.
- **Vitamin A**: (Beta-Carotene–2400 mg/day) It is required for clear vision and healthy skin. Excess of vitamin A leads to toxicity and can be harmful. Vitamin A level in the body can be maintained by consuming oranges, carrots, vegetables (green and leafy ones), fruits (mango, papaya and tomato) and whole milk.
- **Vitamin D**: This is synthesised through sunlight which aids in the absorption of calcium in the body.
- **Iodine**: This has to be maintained in the body by adequate diet containing iodine. Natural sources of iodine are cereals, nuts, and oil seeds. These are rich in iodine mineral.

Yoga and slimming

Organ	Recommended Yoga Postures
For slimming back	Halasana, Paschimottanasana, Shalabhasana, Virbhadrasana.
Fatness on hips	Konasana, Halasana, Janusirasana, Vajroli Mudra, Mayurasana, Natrajasana.
Fat around stomach/trunk	Supta Vajrasana, Natrajasana, Mayurasana
To slim the abdomen	Yog Mudra, Paschimottanasana, Shalabhasana, Mayurasana.
Slimming of legs, kness and thighs	Meditation, Supta Vajrasana, Virbhadrasana, Ardha Chandrasana and Trikonasana.
To trim arms, hands/wrists	Mayurasana, Janusirasana.
To trim spinal column	Ardha Chandrasana, Halasana, Bhujangasana, Natrajasana.
Slimming the whole body	Mayurasana, Dhanurasana, Natrajasana.

Given below are a few Yoga exercises suitable for slimming the whole body:

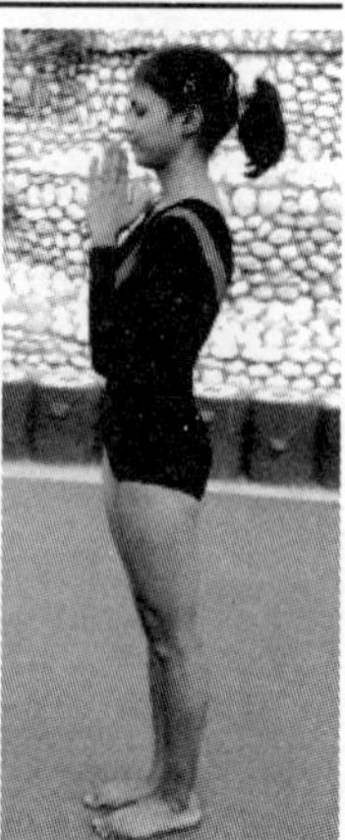

Sun exercise (surya namaskarasana)

This *asana* involves various bending forward and backward postures. It comprises the following benefits:

- The *asana* slims and trims the whole body.
- It stretches all the abdominal organs and improves digestion.
- It activates all the glands of the endocrinal system (the pancreas, adrenal, thyroid, pituitary and some other glands begin to secrete their respective hormones).

- This *asana* invigorates the facial tissues, the central nervous system and all the organs of the upper part of the body.
- It also tones the liver and massages the kidneys and adrenal glands.
- It develops the chest and exercises the spine between the shoulder blades and makes them more active, efficient and healthy.

Practice of the Sun Exercise

1. Stand erect with legs together, arms on sides. This is *Tadasana.* Place the palms together in front of the chest in *Namaskar mudra.* Keep the eyes closed, relax the whole body and breathe normally.
2. Raise both the arms upwards, inhale slowly. Stretch and bend downward to touch the floor with both the hands.
3. Finish exhaling. Put both hands on the floor. Raise your head and stretch the left leg backward.

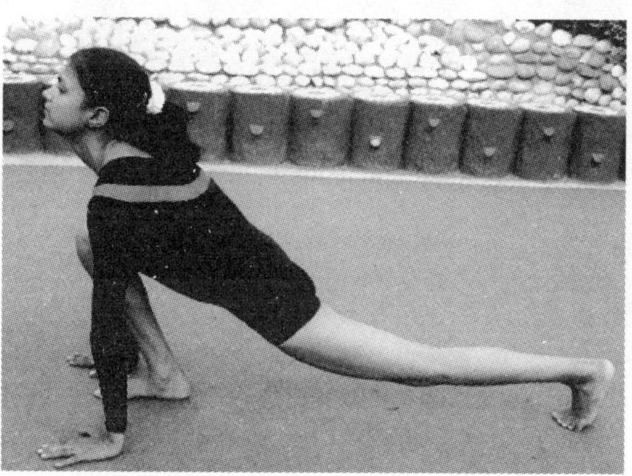

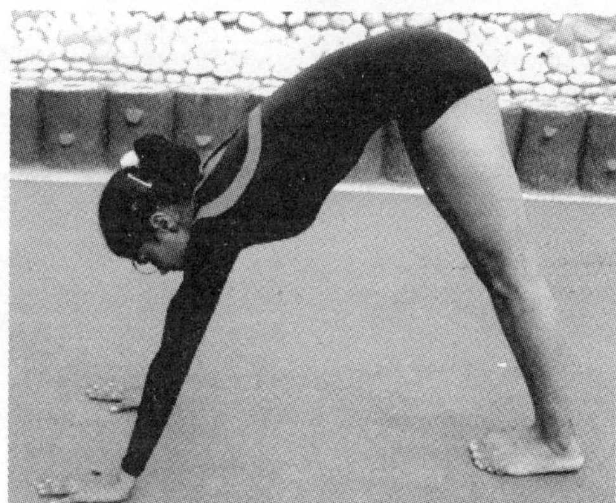

4. Stretch the right leg too and raise the body.
5. Lower the chest and touch the floor with your chin.

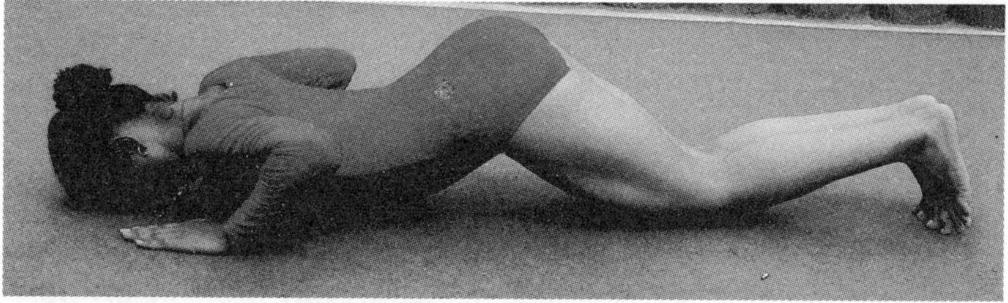

6. Raise your head, trunk, hips, thighs and knees from the floor.
7. Bring your right foot forward and stretch back the left leg.

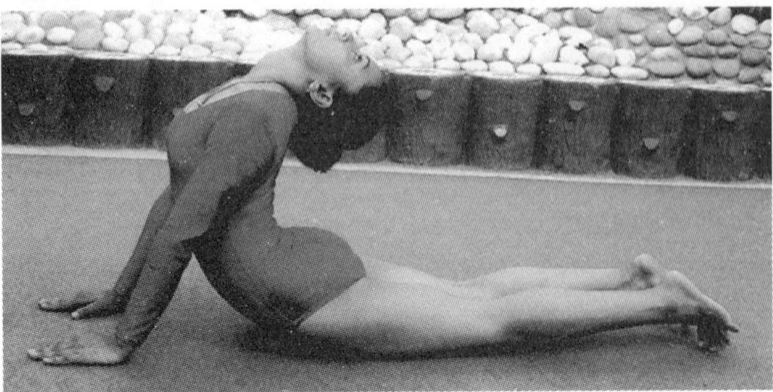

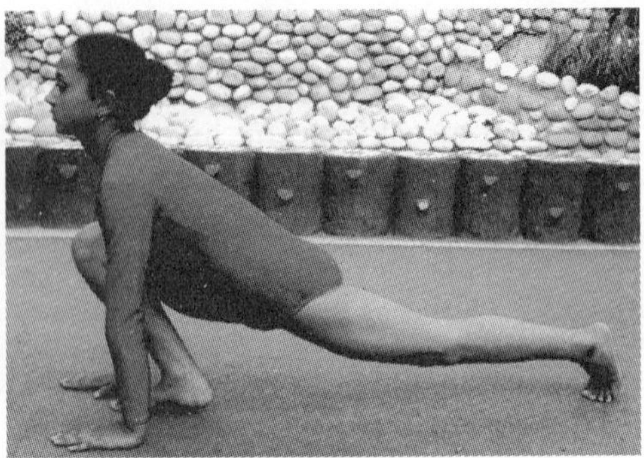

8. Raise the body with your hands backwards.
9. Bend backwards with raised hands and feet joined.

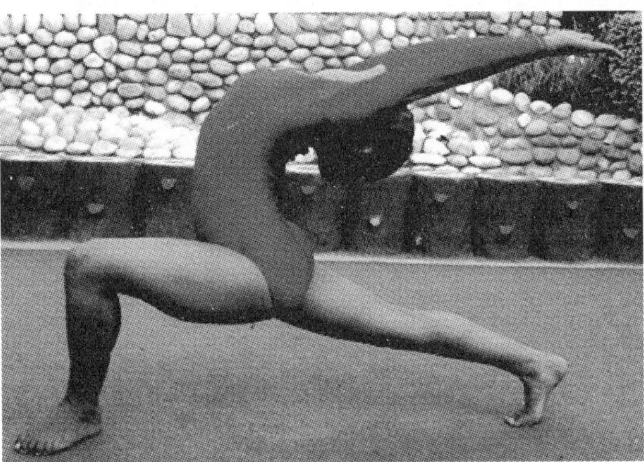

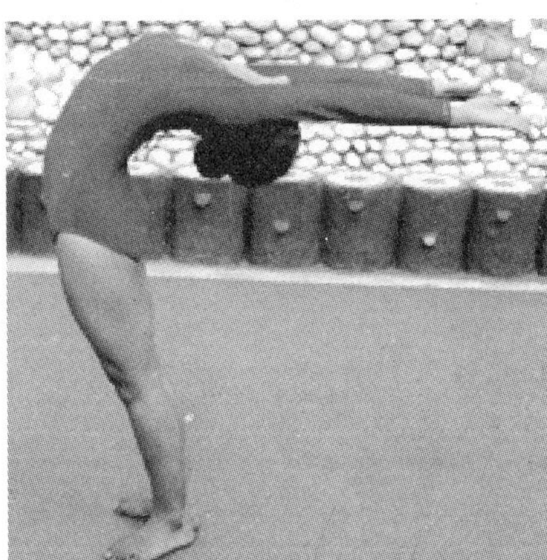

10. Return to the original position, standing with folded hands.

Precautions: Avoid the practice of *Surya Namaskarasana* in case of:

- Severe high blood pressure.
- A heart disease.
- Epilepsy, hernia, slip disc and spondylosis.
- Menstrual periods.
- Advanced stage of pregnancy.

Mayurasana (peacock posture)

Kneel on the ground, knees apart and palms flat on the floor. Now bring the elbows under the abdomen just below the navel. Lean forward to touch the ground with forehead and stretch out the legs with feet raised. Raise head and keep the body horizontally parallel to the ground. Stay balanced on the arms as long as possible. Lie down on the stomach, relax for some time breathing normally. Repeat the *asana* two to three times.

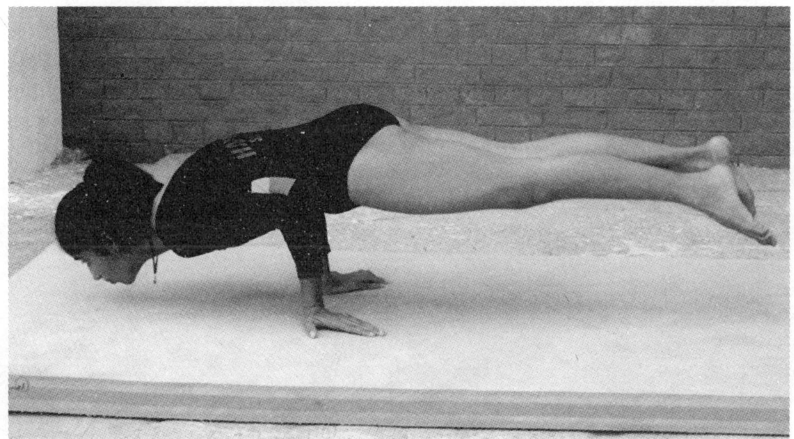

Benefits

- It is an *asana* to slim the whole body and it increases the supply of blood to the digestive organs. If it is carried out in an incorrect manner, it can lead to chronic constipation and result in faulty digestive system.
- It tones up the abdominal muscles and brings the body into equilibrium.
- It strengthens the muscles of the hands, wrists and forearms.
- It stimulates the muscles around the anus and the lower part of the trunk.
- Regenerates the sexual glands and is a useful *asana* for those teenagers suffering from emission.

Precautions: Always perform this posture with the lungs empty.

Vajroli mudra (boat posture)

This is a balancing pose which strengthens and slims the thighs and the abdominal muscles. This *asana* rids the digestive organs of toxins and helps to develop sexual willpower in men and women between the age of 25–40.

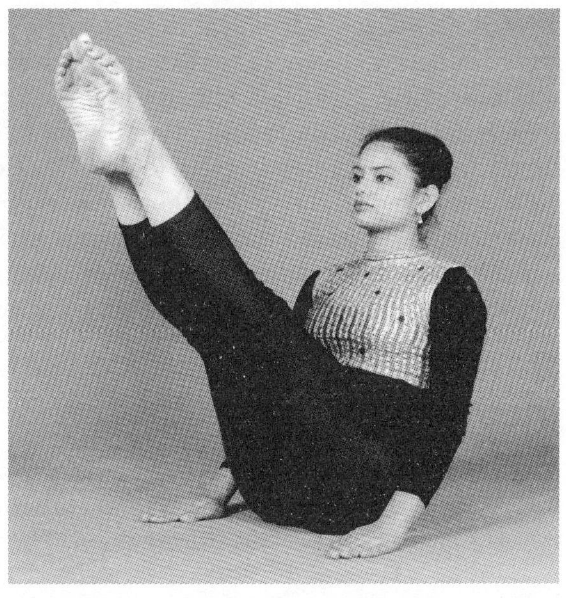

Matsyasana (fish posture)

Sit in *Padmasana.* Lean the trunk backwards with the help of elbows. Lift the chest upwards resting the crown of your head on the floor. Hold the posture for one to two minutes, then return to the starting position. Relax lying on the back and repeat this exercise three to four times.

This is a posture beneficial for the entire body. It strengthens the spinal column, provokes an abundant flow of blood to all the organs of the body, fortifies the back muscles, keeps the abdominal organs healthy, refreshes the body and mind, removes aches and stiffness, stretches the neck muscles and renders it supple.

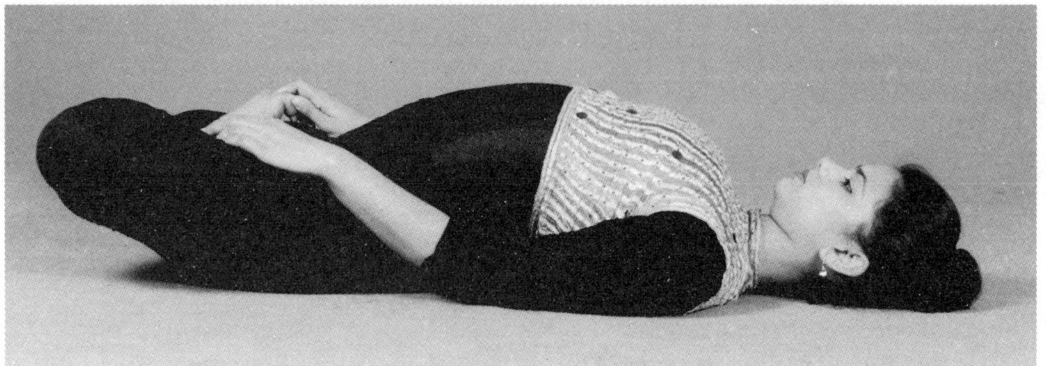

Natarajasana

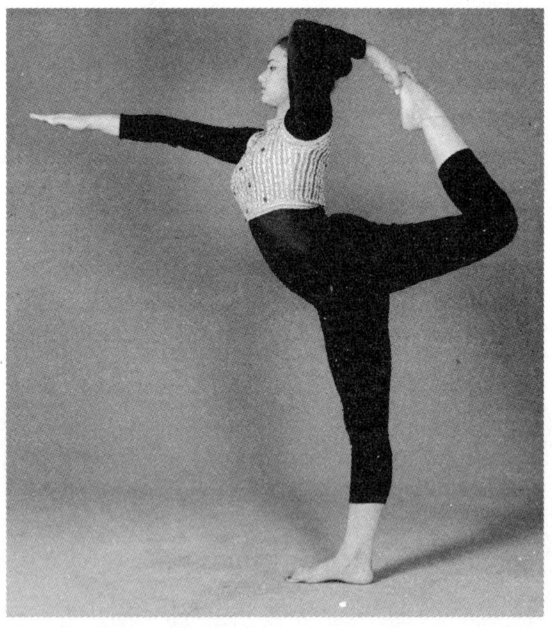

'Nataraj' posture is dedicated to **Lord Shiva**. As a cosmic dancer, Shiva is called the *God of dance.* This posture generates vigour, vitality, potency and beauty, flexibility to the limbs, shoulders and hip joints, strengthens the major bones of the body, enhances digestive power, leaves a good effect upon the spine and has a slimming effect on most of the organs of the body.

To practise *Natarajasana,* stand up on the left leg. Fold back the right leg at the knee and grab the toes of the right leg with the palm of the right hand. Now tighten and raise the left hand slowly in front pushing the right foot backwards. Now bend the body above the waist slightly forward and try to see the finger of your raised hand. Stay in this position for about eight seconds breathing normally. Return to the initial position and repeat the posture on the other side. Make four to six rounds daily.

Mud therapy

Earth was used extensively for remedial purposes in ancient times. In modern times, it again has come into prominence as a valuable therapeutic agent. Earth has remarkable effects upon the human body, especially during night. These effects are described as refreshing, invigorating and vitalising. For wounds and skin diseases, application of clay or moistened earth is a natural bandage.

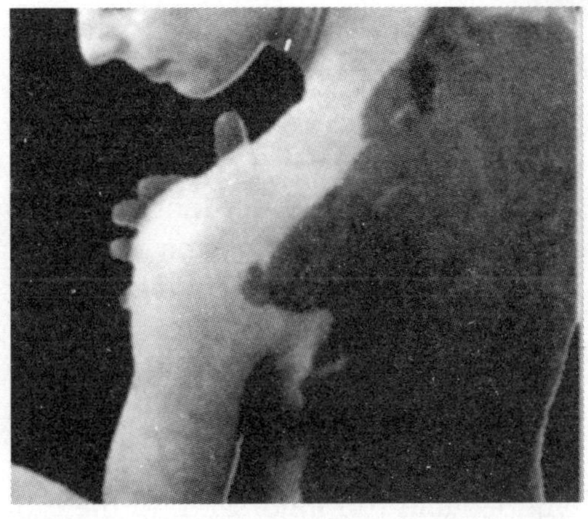

The healing power of earth is very strong as compared to the leaves and herbs. The precious gift from the womb of the earth not only refreshes, invigorates and revitalises the skin but also helps in curing chronic inflammation caused by internal disease, bruises, sprains, boils and sunburn. The cold moisture in the mud packs relaxes the skin pores, draws blood into the surface, relieves congestion and pain, besides promoting heat radiation. A mud pack is prepared with clay obtained from about six feet below the surface of the earth ensuring that it does not contain impurities such as dust particles or pebbles. The clay is then made into a smooth paste with warm water. It is then allowed to cool for a while before applying on the body.

Application of Mud Bandage: It is a beneficial treatment, if applied:

- **On the head:** Cures headache, hypertension, mental tension and sleeplessness.
- **On the spinal cord:** It has beneficial effect on the psychic centre, strengthens the nerve system of the brain, cures mental tension, anaemia, pregnancy disorders, male impotency (mud bandage applied on male organ), frigidity among women (mud bandage applied on lower abdomen) and obesity.
- **On eyes:** This has beneficial effect on weak eyesight, dark circles around the eyes, watery eyes, glaucoma and puffy eyes.
- **On ears:** It cures pus discharge, inflammation and pain if the mud pack is applied around the ears. If the condition is severe, mix *neem* water or potassium permanganate or epsom salt in the mud.
- **On the breats:** Rub your breasts with dry towel to stimulate the blood circulation in muscles. Apply mud bandage (not over 15 minutes). It helps to cure lung disorders and development of (over-developed or under-developed) breasts.
- **On abdomen and waistline:** It cures kidney disorders, dysentery, uterus disorders, menstruation problems and fatness around the waist.
- **On female sex organs:** It helps in the treatment of gynaecological disorders and scanty and painful menstruation discharge, profuse bleeding, irregular periods, leucorrhoea (white discharge laced with pus), spotting blood in urine, itching at the vaginal skin and vaginal odour.

The mud bath

The mud bath is found to tone up the skin by increasing the blood circulation and energising the skin tissues. Frequent mud bath improves the complexion, clears spots and patches on the skin and treats skin diseases like psoriasis. However, the duration of a mud bath should be about 30–45 minutes.

Sleeping on the earth

Make a sand bed 6 feet long, 3 feet wide and 6 inches thick in a pollution-free and calm atmosphere. Sleeping on the mud or sand bed for 3-4 hours equalises 8 hours of sleep on the bed. Make sure to remove your clothes before lying on the sand bed. The treatment is useful for curing mental tension, body pain, skin diseases, epilepsy, tiredness, hypertension, heart disease, anaemia and depression.

Mud-sand bath

Undress and rub mud/sand (in the ratio of 60:40) on your abdomen, breasts, legs, arms and other parts of the body. Do a light exercise before taking bath and rub your body with dry towel to produce heat. Do not eat anything for about four hours prior to taking this kind of bath. Massage at night with coconut, *arandi* or *mahua* oil or *desi ghee.* This technique cures body itch, high blood pressure, body odour, skin disorders (e.g. leucoderma, pityriasis, urticaria and eczema).

Massage with aromatic oils

Essential oils are highly volatile, evaporating readily on exposure to air and when inhaled may enter the body. When diluted and applied externally, essential molecules enter the skin. Both the treatments enable you to inhale and absorb the oils. All essential oils appear to be antiseptic and bactericidal to some diseases and are helpful in the treatment of viral infection. Massage with essential oils is very useful for the skin, vigour and vitality. Use a light vegetable oil scented with a few drops of essential oil for massage. Do not pour the oil directly on to the body. Pour about a teaspoon of oil into the palm, then rub your hands together to warm them slightly and massage. Essential oils, blended with massage oil, add a new dimension to massage and impart a feeling of luxury to the massage. The perfume in the oil can help to relax or refresh. Essential oils have many properties, e.g., some are anti-bacterial, others are antiseptic or anti-inflammatory.

Aromatherapy is the practice of using aromatic oils therapeutically to treat many skin problems, e.g., acne, scars and ageing besides disorders, e.g., stress, insomnia, mental depression and nervous tension. Essential oils are extremely concentrated and must be diluted in a carrier oil while using them, otherwise they can cause allergies. The most common carrier oils are almond, soya, grape-seed, avocado, peach and wheat-germ oils. To dilute an essential oil, one to three drops are mixed with five teaspoons of carrier oil. Bergamot oil has antiseptic, astringent properties and is used for acne, greasy skin and hair treatments. Chamomile possesses calming, soothing effect and is used for sensitive skins. Clary sage has astringent, stimulating properties and used as a fixative. Eucalyptus, with antiseptic stimulating properties, is capable of treat aches and pains. Frankincense, having calming, relaxing properties, combats wrinkles on the skin. Neroli has sedative, aphrodisiac, analgesic, calming properties and is suitable for dry skin. Rose possesses antiseptic, sedative, depressant properties and is very useful for all types of skins. Sandalwood has antiseptic, sedative, calming, aphrodisiac properties and treats dry, dehydrated and acne skins. Tea tree oil with antiseptic, germicidal, fungicidal, soothing, healing properties treats infections, pimples, boils and burns. Ylang Ylang has anti-depressant, sedative, antiseptic, aphrodisiac properties and cures skin problems. It is especially good for oily skins.

Basic essential oil facial massage movements include massaging and pressing various reflex points, carrying out various light effleurage and deeper tissue movements on both sides of the face, neck and shoulders. Warm your hands by rubbing them together with light friction and imagine warm energy flowing into them. Pour a little massage oil into the palm of a hand and rub both the hands together. Start at the chin and work up the face, massage in sections towards the forehead. Gently place hands on the muscle and move towards the occipital bone in a continuous flowing movement. Start with the right hand, followed by the left hand. Pour a little of the massage oil into your hands and use light effleurage movements upwards over the face with small circular travelling movements with the middle finger. Start at the centre of the upper lip on the face, work towards the ear and the whole area under the lower lip with gentle pressure, small circular, stationary movements. Take cheek muscle between your thumbs and index fingers, and gently squeeze moving underneath the cheekbone. Rest for five seconds, with both hands on the face. The movement aids the flow of energy.

Aroma massage

There are three ways in which essential oil molecules enter the body and leave an effect on it—by *inhalation*, by *trans-dermal absorption* and by *ingestion*. In general sense, aromatherapy increases the blood supply to the tissues, which helps the proliferation of cells and regeneration, increasing oxygenation and lymphatic flow. The body massage treatments using essential oils can be for slimming, toning, energising, relaxing and healing.

There are several reflex points on the body. Finger pressure is applied by placing the middle finger over the index finger, and using the lower finger to massage the reflex points with small, stationary, circular movements. Stationary indicates that the fingertip does not move over the skin but stays at one reflex point, moving in small circles. The pressure should not be applied for more than three seconds at each point. The important pressure points (reflex points) on the body are:

- The sole of the foot which energises and stimulates the whole body.
- Pressing on the back, at about one inch above or two inches on the waistline level and on either side of the vertebrae energises and stimulates the entire body. Pressing on the front, about three inches below and one inch either side of the navel helps weight reduction, cellulite and improves circulation and reproduction system. This stimulates and energises the body, especially the abdominal area.
- If the face looks tired or is sagging, apply pressure at the centre of the cheekbone on both sides of the face.

- Massaging on either side of the nose and on inner corners of the eyes helps to reduce puffy eyes.
- Apply pressure on the face at the outer corners of the eyes, in case the face looks tired or is sagging.
- Massage on both sides on the face, in the hollows just below the ears, helps droopy cheeks and jowls.
- Massage on both sides of the face between eye sockets and cheekbones helps reducing eye bags.

Symptoms that appear in a female with advancing age

The brain starts maturing rapidly by the age of three. The sex hormones start producing in the female body by the age of seven. The growth accelerates up to the age of puberty and starts to slow down until long bones stop growing by the age of twenty. A female becomes hyper fertile in the early twenties, followed by a decline in her fertility till she reaches the age of thirty. The height of a female starts to diminish gradually between the age of thirty to forty. The hair pigment cells in the scalp start reducing their activities between the age of forty to fifty. Lot of care is needed between the age of fifty to sixty, when the body may begin to put on weight during the period of menopause. From the age between sixty to seventy, the red blood cells start reducing in the body and the quality of the skin begins to deteriorate. In the age group of seventy to eighty, the spine starts to curve as the spinal disc shrinks and bones in a female body become thinner and weaker. Between the age of eighty to ninety, the body loses seventy percent of the muscle mass as compared to her youth.

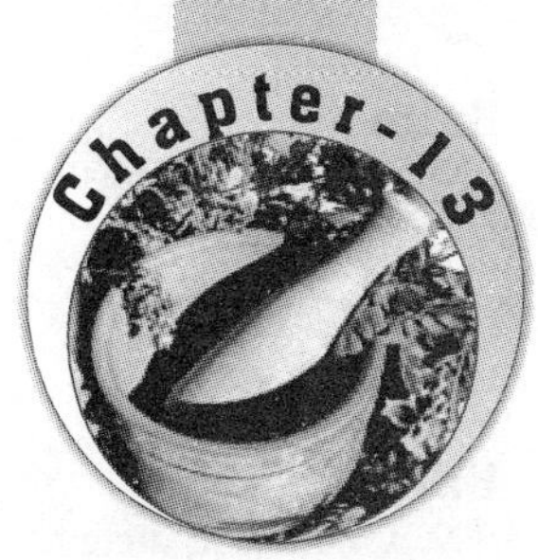

Herbs with Cosmetic Applications

Abbreviations BN: Botanical Name F: Family

Common Name	Description
Aloe Extract *(Gwarpatha)* F : Liliaceae	Aloe, commonly known as *Kumari* or *Kanya* (means virgin girl), has been used in medicines and cosmetics since the time of Greeks and Egyptians, and believed to have been used by Cleopatra to keep the complexion clear and soft. Aloe vera is used in cosmetic preparations due to its softness, tenderness, moisturising, soothing and calming properties. It is excellent for dry and sensitive skins as well as for the treatment of sunburns and other minor burns, insect bites and skin irritations. Aloe vera is an emollient with hydrating, softening, moisturising, healing, anti-microbial and anti-inflammatory properties. It penetrates the skin, supplying moisture directly to the tissue and absorbs UV light. It has effect on the skin, making it beneficial for sensitive, dry, sunburned and sun-exposed skins.
Arnica Extract BN:Arnica Montana	A botanical herb credited with a wide variety of properties including antiseptic, astringent, anti-microbial, anti-inflammatory, anti-coagulant, circulation-stimulating and healing. It is considered excellent for an acne condition. It is effective in gels and creams designed to treat damaged, reddened or tired skin. The extract is obtained from the flowers.
Avocado Oil F : Laurace	This oil is obtained from the ripe avocado fruit and from the seed. Rich and nourishing with high vitamin content, the pulp is used in face masks and the oil in nourishing creams. Avocado oil is used as an emollient and a carrier oil in a cosmetic preparations. Its skin-benefiting properties include bactericidal and soothing to sensitive skin, increases the collagen of connective tissue and keeps the skin moist and smooth. In cosmetic formulations, it is effectively used in cleansing creams, moisturisers, lipsticks, make-up bases, bath oils, sunscreen and suntan preparations.

Balm
BN: Melissa Officinalis
F : Labiatae

A fragrant woodland plant with dark green wrinkled leaves and small creamy flowers. It helps in the treatment of eczema, dry skin, acne and blemished (sensitive) skins. The balm attributes calming, soothing, healing, antispasmodic, tightening, anti-bacterial, and circulation stimulating properties.

Basil *(Tulsi)*
BN: Ocimum Sanctum Linn
F : Labiatae

An aromatic herb with white flowers and oval shaped, shiny leaves. Medicinally, basil is a potent tonic having both stimulant and nervine effect. It is particularly good at arresting morning and travel sickness. Basil oil often used as a carrier oil, has stimulating, tonic, purifying, anti-bacterial and anti-microbial properties. It has application in acne preparations.

Blackberry *(Jamun)*

Berries are delicious, extraordinarily rich in vitamin C, but leaves are mildly aperient and accredited with sound tonic virtues which can also be applied externally as a lotion to cure psoriasis and scaly conditions of the skin. Its astringent and tonic properties can be beneficially used for acne conditions.

Birch *(Bhojpatra)*
Betula alba Linn proparte

An astringent, antiseptic, softening, circulation stimulating herb. Birch has curative properties in case of skin diseases such as acne, eczema, sunburn and hair loss.

Borage
(Pathharchoor)
BN: Coleus amboinicus
F : Labiatae

Borage has beneficial effect on heart, kidneys, adrenal glands and the entire digestive system. It cures allergic reactions and ringworm when applied direct to the skin. Borage is an effective anti-irritant and has hydrating properties.

Bergamot *(Zabir)*

An aromatic herb, used to prepare perfumes, colognes and toilet waters and helps tanning. Bergamot oil is considered an antiseptic and bacterial growth inhabitor, considered good for oily and acne skin and for seborrhoeic conditions. Exposure to sun after applying bergamot oil may cause hyperpigmentation and a skin rash.

Carrot Oil
(Gajar Ka Tel)
BN : Daucus
F : Umbelliferae

Derived from the carrot root, carrot oil is used since the 16th century for skin diseases due to its believed cleansing, depurative and draining properties. The herb has been indicated for acne skin conditions, dermatitis, skin irritation, skin rashes and wrinkles.

Calendula *(Genda)*
BN : Marigold
F : Compositae

The flowers and leaves are very beneficial for clearing the skin of eczema, spots and grease. It is claimed to be rejuvenating. It is an emollient said to have healing, soothing, antispetic, anti-itching and anti-inflammatory properties.

Comfrey
BN : Symphytum
F : Boraginaceae

A plant with healing, astringent, and emollient properties. It is used in case of itching, swelling, bruising, cuts, papules and pustules besides curing eczema and sunburns.

Celandine

The herb plant is found in hedgerows and wastes, with yellowish hairy leaves shaped like the oak leaves and yellow flowers. As a wart cure, the raw yellow juice should be applied direct to the skin.

Cleavers

The plant has tiny white flowers and small round fruits. The herb is an excellent remedy for the scalp and the skin. It clears dandruff, cures leprosy and skin cancer. Cleavers extract is said to be useful in treating eczema and spots and is recommended for normal to dry skins.

Clove *(Laung)*
F : Myriaceae

An aromatic spice used in skin tonics and stimulating face masks. It has powerful, antiseptic, cicatrizant properties with a strong germicidal effect.

Chamomile

Has daisy-like flowers and feathery grey green leaves, usually found in waste places. An infusion of leaves and flowers of this plant, fresh or dried, has a wide variety of cosmetic and medicinal uses. Anti-allergic, healing, cooling, analgesic and antiseptic agent, chamomile dissolves tumours, heals ulcers, expels worms, banishes tiredness, treats many female disorders. As a cosmetic, the herb can be used as a face-wash to clarify complexion, cure dermatitis and as a rinse to lighten fair hair.

Dandelion *(Dulal/Dudhal/Kanphool)*
F : Asteraceae

The golden-yellow flower head of the plant has several medicinal values. It is widely used to cure pimples, acne and skin spots, refreshes the skin, corrects pH balance, increases the respiratory capacity of the skin tissues and is beneficial for dry skins. The plant root is used for cosmetic preparations rather than the flower, as juice of the root is the more powerful part of the plant.

Elder
BN : Sambucus Linn
F : Caprifoliaceae

All parts of the tree are used. Its leaves, combined with honey, is a standard infusion that clears problem or inflamed skin. It soothes all burns and scalds and is beneficial for treating dry skin. A balm of elder flowers keeps crow's feet at bay. The herb has astringent, antiseptic, emollient cooling properties. In the 19th century, elder flower water was commonly used to clear the complexion of freckles and sunburn, and keep the skin in good condition.

Emblica Gaetrn *(Amla)* F : Euphorbiaceae

An astringent herb, rich source of vitamin C and useful for hair and skin treatment.

Fennel *(Saunf)*
BN : Foeniculum Mill
F : Umbelliferae

The herb has a cleansing effect on the skin. It is beneficial for the oily skin types. When steaming the face, use it in the water.

Garlic *(Lehsun)*

Recognised as an antiseptic and bactericide, garlic ointment applied externally reduces hard swelling and is useful for treating problem skins including acne and eczema.

Henna *(Mehendi)*
F : Lythraceae

An astringent and antiseptic herb with cooling properties used for hair conditioning, hair dye and for applying over hands and feet. Primarily, it is a colourant that provides a reddish brown shade. Generally, the extract is obtained from the leaves.

Horse Radish Extract
BN : Cochlearia
F : Cruciferae

Traditionally used against sunburns, superficial and other nonextensive burns, and to give the skin clarity and freshness. It has antiseptic and skin clearing properties. The extract is made primarily from the plant's roots.

Horsetail extract
BN : Equisetum Linn
F : Equisetaceae

General botanical properties include stimulating, astringent, soothing, healing and softening. The herb regulates the skin, strengthens its connective tissue, prevents and counteracts wrinkles around the eyes and is beneficial in both anti-ageing and acne products.

Hyssop Oil

Properties include healing, tonic and stimulating. It is indicated for dermatitis, eczema and wounds.

Ivy Extract *(Lablab)*
F : Araliaceae

Ivy extract is said to have a slimming and anti-cellulite effect due to its ability to prevent water accumulation in the skin tissue. It has soothing, anti-bacterial, anti-parasitic, decongestant and analgesic properties. Ivy leaves are traditionally used to treat various skin eruptions and skin ulcers.

Jasmine Oil
(Chameli Ka Tel)
BN : Jasminum Officinale

A highly aromatic oil made from the flowers and used as a perfume in many recipes. The oil is credited with moisturising, soothing and healing properties. It is ideal for dry and sensitive skins and cures dermatitis.

Jatropha Curcas
(Ratanjot, Jangli Arand, Safed Arand)
F : Euphorbiaceae

The herb is said to have cleaning, stimulating and haemostatic action. The oil obtained from seeds is very effective against scabies, eczema and dermatitis. The root bark is used as an external application for sores. The oil is applied to hair as growth stimulator. The tender twigs of plant are used for cleaning teeth and relieve toothache and strengthen gums.

Indian Sarsaparilla
(Hindisalsa, Sariwa)
BN : Hemidesmus indicus
F : Asclepiadaceae

The herb has deodorant, anti-itch action. The roots are claimed to cure leucoderma, itching, several other skin diseases and foul odour from the body. A gargle of the herb is good for toothache and decay.

Juniper Oil
(Hauber/Huber)
F : Coniferae

Has antiseptic, astringent, cleansing and toning properties. It is considered helpful in treating acne, excessive oily skin, dermatitis and eczema.

Lavender
BN : Lavendula vera
F : Labiatae

It has a pleasant fragrance and is used for scenting bath water. Lavender is also used as gargle or mouth wash. The oil is credited with many properties which include anti-allergic, anti-inflammatory, antiseptic, anti-bacterial, anti-spasmodic, balancing, energising, soothing, healing, tonic and stimulating. Lavendar oil works well on all types of skins and produces excellent results when used for oily skin as well as in the treatment of acne, burns, dermatitis, eczema and psoriasis.

Lettuce *(Salad Patta)*
BN : Lactuca F : Asteraceae

Rich in minerals, iron and vitamins. It is cooling and excellent for sunburn, skin inflammation and redness.

Marigold
(Genda flower)

It is a disinfectant herb used in effective treatment of ulcers and open sores. The plant cures varicose veins and other circulatory troubles. Marigold infusion (petals only) provides the ideal balancer of an over-oily skin and all complexions. It has antiseptic, healing and soothing effect and heals sunburns and skin rashes.

Mint *(Pudina)*

It has cooling, tonic, stimulating, antiseptic and relaxing properties. This aromatic herb is widely used as a fragrance in beauty products, serves as a cleanser for acne and dermatitis treatment.

Myrrh *(Bol/Beajabol)*
F : Burseraceae

It is said to have disinfectant, antiseptic, anti-inflammatory, anti-itching, cicatrizant, tonic, stimulant, sedative and astringent properties. The extract can be valuable in products designed for acne treatment and was used by ancient Egyptian women in facial masks and other cosmetic preparations.

Myrtle
(Vilayati Mehendi)
F : Mystaceae

It is astringent and antiseptic with botanical properties closely resembling those of eucalyptus. Useful for acne and oily skin.

Nettle *(Bichoobooti)*
BN : Geleopsis
F : Urticaceae

Its botanical properties include as anti-inflammatory, astringent, bactericidal, healing, mildly deodorant, antioxidant and stimulating, rich in vitamin E. It is effective for treating eczema and sunburn.

Oat

The extract, obtained from the seeds of oats, has soothing properties on the skin. It enhances emulsion stability, increases viscosity, leaves a smooth afterfeel and provides a source of whole natural vegetable protein. It cures irritated skins resulting from sunburn, psoriasis, allergic dermatitis, relieves redness and itching. Oats in the form of bran, flour, or meal provide a gentle base for face masks for delicate, sensitive skin.

Olive Oil
(Jaitun Ka Tel)

A pale colour carrier oil with excellent lubricity and low odour. Olive leaf extract possesses astringent, antiseptic, antioxidant and vasodilatant properties. It is used in anti-ageing products.

Orange Flower Oil
(Narangi Ka Tel)
F : Rutaceae

It is credited with soothing and calming properties when used in skin care preparations.

Peppermint
F : Labiate

Credited with refreshing, cooling, bactericidal and anti-irritant properties. The herb helps relieve skin irritation, itching and skin redness due to inflammation or acne.

Rose *(Gulab)*
BN : Rosa Linn
F : Rosaceae

Rose extract is credited with astringent, tonic and deodorant properties. Rose oil has been credited with antiseptic, disinfectant, slightly tonic, soothing and moisturising properties. It may be beneficial to all skin types, particularly mature, dry or sensitive skins. Rosewater is credited with soothing, cooling, moisturising, astringent and cleansing properties when applied to abrasions and other superficial skin lesions. A cellular stimulant and tissue regenerator, rosewater is beneficial to sensitive, wrinkled and aged skin.

Rosemary *(Rusmari)*
BN : Rosemarianus Linn
F : Labiatae

A popular garden plant with spiky dark green leaves and distinctive scent. As a cosmetic ingredient, rosemary is a fine tonic for the scalp and skin. It adds lustre to the hair, is a common ingredient of many commercial shampoos, keeps the skin free from wrinkles and youth alive. Rosemary extract has astringent, toning, stimulating, deodorant, antiseptic, reactivating, anti-bacterial, softening and invigorating properties. It helps improve skin regeneration. Rosemary oil is credited with antiseptic properties and is considered beneficial for acne, dermatitis and eczema.

Sage *(Safakuss)*
BN : Salvia officinalis
F : Labiatae

An aromatic, sun-loving plant with grey green leaves and mauvish flowers. Sage oil is credited with depurative and healing properties and indicated for acne and oily skin. Sage extract is considered to have astringent, invigorating and healing properties. It is used as a remedy for every type of inflammation.

Sandalwood oil
(Chandan Ka Tel)
F : Santalaceae

It is usually credited with astringent, anti-inflammatory, anti-bacterial, tonic, stimulant, cooling and soothing properties. It is a good antiseptic in case of acne and an astringent for oily skin.

Sesame Oil *(Til)*
F : Pedaliaceae

Commonly used as a carrier oil for cosmetic products and has emollient properties. Sesame oil is useful in suntan lotions and blocks 30 percent of the sun's burning UV rays.

Shikakai *(Kochi)*
BN : Acacia Concinna

Used to remove dandruff and cure skin diseases. Extensively used as a detergent for washing hair.

Soapwart Extract
BN : Yucca Linn
F : Agavaceae

It is credited with cleansing properties and due to its saponin content, it is also said to be soothing to the skin and to relieve itching. In traditional medicine, soapwart extract is used for treating acne, psoriasis and eczema. The extract is made from the roots of the plant, though the leaves and stem may also be used.

Soap Nut Tree
(Reetha)
BN : Spindus Linn
F : Sapindaceae

Used as detergent for washing hair because of its cleansing action. Fruits/Seeds are used to cure pimples and scabies.

Strawberry
BN : Fragaria F : Rosaceae

Strawberry juice can be used to treat more serious skin ailments such as eczema, pruritis and sunburnt skins.

Tea Tree Oil

Has antiseptic, germicidal and expectorant properties. Pale, yellow to colourless oil is credited to heal skin disorders and infections, to fight against seborrhoea, psoriasis, acne, scaling and redness of skin, eczema, itching and dermatitis, The oil is ideal for aromatherapy given its low toxicity.

Turmeric *(Haldi)*
BN : Curcuma Linn
F : Zingiberaceae

It is credited with healing, tonic, mildly stimulating, anti-inflammatory, skin softening and blood-purifying properties. The herb is useful for a variety of curative purposes including the treatment of eczema, acne, skin infections, ulcers, burns and rashes.

Vervain *(Holywort)*
BN : Verbena Linn
F : Verbenaceae

Green-grey leaves and small-hooded mauve flowers of the plant has properties to cure several health disorders, relieves mental strain, helps cure infectious diseases of skin.

Walnut *(Akhrot)*
F : Jaglandaceae

Traditionally used herb known for its soothing, fungistatic and astringent, anti-itching properties. It can be used in case of sunburns, acne and other skin diseases. The extract is obtained from the leaves and bark, and the oil is extracted from the ripe nut.

Witchhazel
BN : Hamamelis
F : Hamamelidaeae

Traditionally used in topical treatment of burns, sunburns and skin irritation because of its anti-inflammatory, anti-itching, softening, emollient and wound healing properties.

Yarrow *(Gandana)*
BN : Achillea Linn
F : Compositae

A plant having greyish, feathery, ethereal-looking leaves and clusters of small daisy-like flowers is considered good in the case of oily and acne skin, because of having astringent, antiseptic, anti-inflammatory, healing and calming properties.

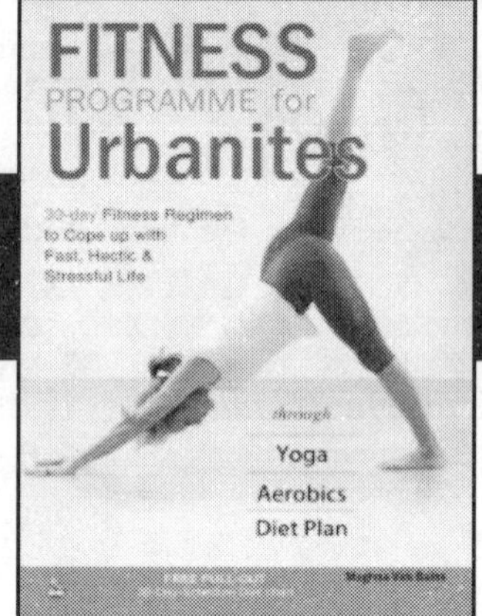

Fitness Programme for Urbanites

—Meghna Virk Vains

'Fitness Programme for Urbanites', an intensive 30-day fitness regimen, the book has been custom-made to blend with everyone's preference of exercise regimes. The regime that starts at home is for those who prefer the comfort and familiarity of their own surroundings. Aerobics for those who prefer company while they workout. Swimming for those who wish to combine the benefits of a workout with some fun and fluidity. Gyming for those who enjoy the rigorous workout and like to sweat it out. Finally, yoga for those who prefer not just working on their body but also the mind and the soul. The aim is to help you make the ultimate choice, by learning which of the above fitness activities, used singularly or combined, gives you maximum results. In addition, it gives an in-depth understanding of the importance of working out well, eating and sleeping well, and all the other aspects that make for a truly holistic fitness package. The book, therefore, comprehensively *works towards transformation of one's lifestyle*

Demy Size • Pages: 180
Price: Rs. 150/- • Postage: Rs. 15/-

Home-made Herbal Cosmetics

—*Dr. S. Suresh Babu*

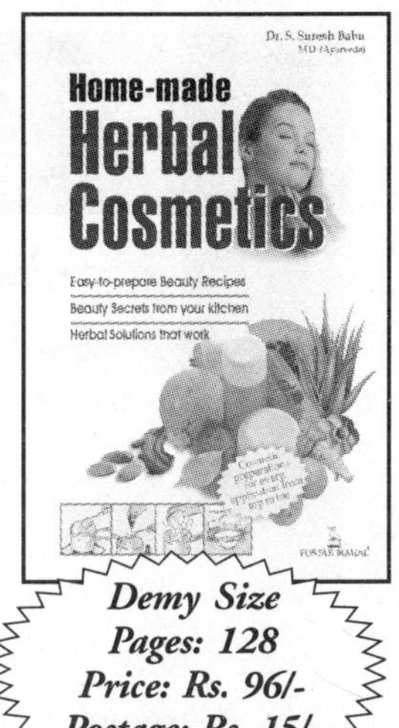

Demy Size
Pages: 128
Price: Rs. 96/-
Postage: Rs. 15/-

The fact that natural herbal products have a definite qualitative edge over chemical-based cosmetics is today universally acknowledged. But then, is every herbal beauty solution as effective as it claims to be? In fact, a lot depends on the extent of knowledge and research put into its preparation.

Home-made Herbal Cosmetics is one such work that brings you herbal solutions that work and work beautifully. Backed by years of research and painstaking effort, it offers comprehensive solutions — from top to toe. For example, castor oil makes an excellent sunscreen — and mixed with a few drops of jasmine oil it becomes a herbal hair conditioner. White wax mixed with almond oil, rose water and sodium benzoate proves effective for dry skin. A mix of pineapple and yoghurt makes an ideal nail soak. Or mineral-rich oatmeal soak has excellent moisturising and softening properties, and serves as a soothing foot bath. The book offers many such formulae and much more.

In addition, there are separate sections devoted to herbal remedies for common ailments (for instance, the milky juice of papaya softens corns, and cotton seed oil applied daily clears spots on the face), and a complete glossary describing the essential qualities and properties of herbal ingredients.

Slim & Smart Body

—*Barun Roy*

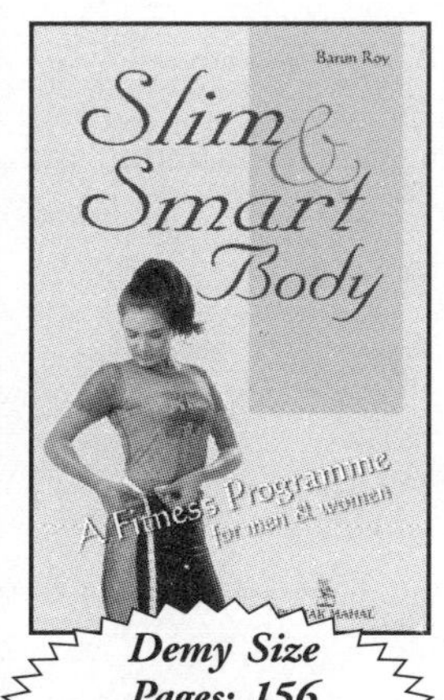

Demy Size
Pages: 156
Price: Rs. 80/-
Postage: Rs. 15/-

Obesity is a worldwide phenomenon with the increasing use of modern gadgets and conveniences, which ensure we do not have to move a muscle except to press the remote button! The burgeoning incidences of disease, depression and premature deaths have meant a rising awareness about the benefits of exercise.

With most exercise regimens making adherents huff and puff, people usually fall by the wayside before the benefits are noticeable. But relax! This book does not expect you to cross the pain barrier. Instead, the focus is on a practical, pleasant and doable exercise regimen where you tailor each programme to suit your individual requirements.

In essence, this book will ensure that exercise is no longer a word you dread, but something you look forward to. The myriad benefits will thereafter flow of their own accord. And a fit, active, healthy life will be your ultimate reward.

Herbal Beauty & Body Care

—Rashmi Sharma

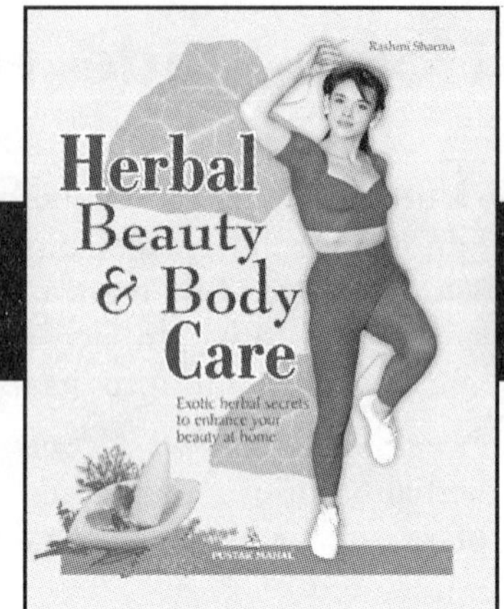

In today's ultra-competitive world, every woman desires to look beautiful. Indeed, well-groomed persons are generally more attractive, strong, poised, outgoing and exciting than poorly groomed people. While modern cosmetics can add a glow to your face and positively enhance the appearance, prolonged exposure to synthetic elements harms your skin. Which is why the world is now recognising the role of herbal products in promoting safe beauty care.

Herbal Beauty Care provides readers with:

- ❖ Synthetic-free easy and effective herbal remedies.
- ❖ Massages and exercises to tone the body.
- ❖ Balanced diet charts.

This is just the book you need for the safe glow that shows in your well-being and appearance.

Big Size • Pages: 144

Price: Rs. **90/-** *• Postage: Rs. 15/- (Also available in Hindi)*

Body & Beauty Care

—Neena Khanna

The image a person projected is of vital importance in career development, opportunity, peer status and ultimate achievement. Poets and artists have long appreciated the crucial role of beauty in human affairs. The latest cosmetic procedures can significantly enhance the appearance of a person.

Body and Beauty Care is primarily intended for the new conscious generation of men and women who groom to look good. Beginning with basic facts about the structure and functioning of the skin, nail, hair and teeth, the book gives the cause and effect of their various problems. It then provides sound advice on the treatment of these problems. A separate chapter deals with modern trends in cosmetic surgery. The book is a must for all those who wish to look good and feel good.

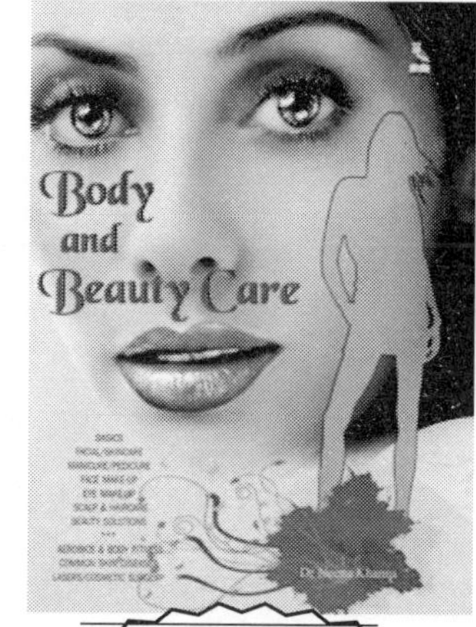

Big Size
Pages: 112
Price: Rs. 120/-
Postage: Rs. 15/-

Home Beauty Clinic

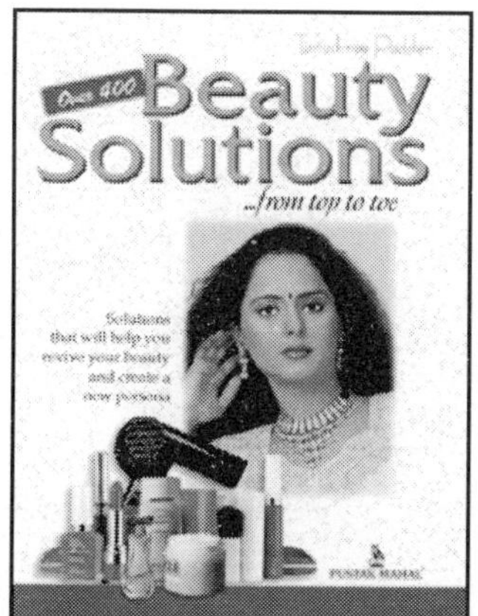

Big Size
Pages: 152
Price: Rs. 150/-
Postage: Rs. 15/-

—Tanushree Podder

Many books have been written on beauty, since this is the biggest obsession with a vast majority of people. But most of these books run along predictable lines and do not fully address the common queries and regular concerns that trouble the minds of men and women. In fact, there is abysmal ignorance and much confusion regarding the basics of hair care, skin care and other related topics.

New terms and products continue to baffle lay minds. This book addresses the long-standing need for authentic information on beauty care. **Over 400 Beauty Solutions** creates proper awareness amongst readers and imparts the latest information on the subject. This is just the right book for every man and woman who wishes to become a beautiful person.